ACUPUNCTURE

for

DENTISTRY

and

OROFACIAL PAIN

GREG GODDARD &
GIOVANNI MAURO

Balboa Press books may be ordered through booksellers or by contacting:

Balboa Press
A Division of Hay House
1663 Liberty Drive
Bloomington, IN 47403
www.balboapress.com
1 (877) 407-4847

ISBN: 978-1-9822-4138-4 (sc)
ISBN: 978-1-9822-4139-1 (e)

Print information available on the last page.

Balboa Press rev. date: 02/04/2020

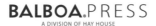

BALBOA.PRESS
A DIVISION OF HAY HOUSE

Contents

Acupuncture for Dentistry and Orofacial Pain

Greg Goddard & Giovanni Mauro

Introduction

Acupuncture strictu sensu is a technique in which practitioners stimulate specific points on the body by inserting thin, flexible needles through the skin. It is one of the practices used in Traditional Chinese Medicine (TCM).

TCM defines acupuncture as the stimulation of specific points on or near the surface of the human body. Any technique of point stimulation can be used, with or without the insertion of needles, including the use of electrical, magnetic, light and sound energy, cupping and moxibustion (the burning on or over the skin of selected herbs), to normalize physiologic functions or to treat various conditions of the human body.

Medicine and dentistry were never considered as separate entities in Eastern cultures as in many European countries since the last century. The two disciplines went through different ways in the US and other Western countries, and this fact determined the lack of knowledge available for the dental professional in the field of acupuncture as a useful tool for dental diseases and orofacial pain.[1]

The scope of the present handbook is to fill this gap. It offers to the dental clinician both a sound and updated knowledge of the theoretical bases of the acupuncture, a discipline that today has gained full recognition. This book will provide the scientific evidence of efficacy and safety in many medical fields, and a comprehensive overview of clinical applications of acupuncture in the different dental areas and orofacial pain.

The present book, based on western scientific evidence, does not imply or assume the recognition in any religion, belief, or 'philosophy.'

Reference

1. Stux G, Pomeranz G. Scientific Basis of Acupuncture: Acupuncture Textbook and Atlas. Heidelberg: Springer Verlag; 1987.

PART 1

THEORETICAL BASIS

1. Traditional Chinese Medicine (TCM) and Acupuncture

TCM is based on ancient concepts, quite distant from conventional Western medicine. TCM includes various forms of herbal medicine, acupuncture, massage (tui na), exercise (qigong), and dietary therapy, but recently also influenced by modern Western medicine.

The doctrines of Chinese medicine are rooted in books such as the Yellow Emperor's Inner Canon and the Treatise on Cold Damage, as well as in cosmological notions such as yin–yang and the five phases.

The description of internal structure and organs in TCM books reads: man is composed of "intestines," the five Tsang, or storing organs, and the six Fu, or eliminating organs.

The five Tsang are the liver, the heart, the spleen, the lungs, the kidneys.

The six Fu are the stomach, the large intestine, the small intestine, the urinary bladder, the gall bladder, and the "three burning spaces"- an imaginary organ, whose three components were held to be distributed over the upper, middle and lower parts of the body.

The storing and eliminating organs are connected by two systems of vessels: those who carry blood and those who carry air or a vital pneuma.

The latter are known as meridians.

Concepts of the body and disease used in TCM reflect its ancient origins and its emphasis on dynamic processes over the physical structure, similar to European humoral theory, where bloodletting and trephination were frequent.

The final endpoint of all the TCM therapies is to restore the so-called qi (pronounced chee), vital energy that flows through meridians, that have branches connected to bodily organs and functions, through complicated pathways embedded throughout the whole body. By stimulating acupuncture points, this flow of energy is harmonized, and optimal health can be restored.

TCM describes health as the harmonious interaction of these entities and the outside world, and disease as a disharmony in interaction. TCM diagnosis aims to trace symptoms to patterns of an underlying disharmony, by measuring the pulse, inspecting the tongue, skin, and eyes, and looking at the eating and sleeping habits of the person as well as many other things.

This holistic approach to a patient, considering the biological, psychological, and social factors as necessary considerations to a successful treatment, is presently gaining acceptance in Western Medicine.[1]

Reference

1. Veith I. Acupuncture in traditional Chinese medicine. An historical review. Calif Med. 1973 Feb;118(2):70-9.

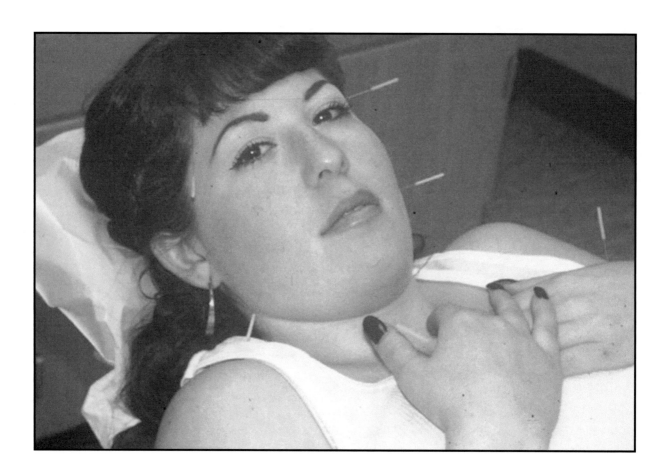

2. Western Evidence Based Acupuncture

The practice of acupuncture to treat identifiable pathophysiological conditions in American medicine was rare until early essays of reciprocal knowledge, back in the 70ies, due to the visit of President Nixon to China in 1972 and the resumption of political, scientific and cultural relations between US and China when there has been an explosion of interest in the United States and Europe in the application of the technique of acupuncture to Western medicine.[1]

Chinese introduced acupuncture as alternative medicine by inserting single nonferromagnetic materials, such as silver or gold, needles at various acupuncture points in the body. At present most of the Chinese acupuncturists recognize stainless surgical steel as the most suitable material for needles, and whatever property was traditionally attributed to precious metals, no differences were noted when using more modern surgical leagues. Chinese acupuncture is traditionally used in a wide range of medical conditions so, when these applications were challenged according to western EBM criteria, various mechanisms were hypothized.[2]

Acupuncture points are the essential components of acupuncture therapy for diagnosis and treatment. Despite numerous studies on defining the significance of acupuncture points from the anatomical or histological perspective, no clear evidence of their existence has been established. Some physiological characteristics of acupuncture points such as tenderness and palpable hardenings are considered as sensitization of nociceptors.[3]

The fundamental theories of acupuncture can be summarized in these three mechanisms:

1. Acupuncture needles can stimulate the afferent nerves (Type I and II) or A-delta fibers which send impulses to the upper centers. At the CNS level, enkephalin and dynorphin are mostly involved in blockage of pain in the spinothalamic tract.

2. Acupuncture stimulates midbrain structures by activating cells in the periaqueductal gray matter and the raphe nucleus. In response, they send descending signals through the dorsolateral tract, causing the release of the monoamines norepinephrine and serotonin in the spinal cord. These neurotransmitters inhibit pain presynaptically and postsynaptically by reducing transmission of signals through the spinothalamic tract. In other terms, acupuncture enhances the descending inhibitory pathways, and modulates the feeling of pain, thus modifying central sensitization. The possible mechanisms underlying the analgesic effects of acupuncture include segmental inhibition and the activation of the endogenous opioid, adrenergic, 5- hydroxytrypyamine, N-metil D-aspartic acid, alpha-amino-3 hydroxy-5 methyl-4 hisoxazolepropionic acid/kainate pathways.

3. Stimulation of pituitary-hypothalamic complex provokes the systemic release of beta-endorphin into the blood, which can result in the release of adrenocorticotropic hormone.[4-6]

Pain is a multidimensional phenomenon. It is among other things, influenced by cognition, context, mood, and many individual differences such as gender or genetic makeup.[7]

References

1. Lewin AJ. Acupuncture and its role in modern medicine. West J Med. 1974 Jan;120(1):27-32.

2. Ceniceros S, Brown GR. Acupuncture: a review of its history, theories, and indications. South Med J. 1998 Dec;91(12):1121-5.

3. Chernyak GV, Sessler DI. Perioperative acupuncture and related techniques. Anesthesiology. 2005;102:1031–49.

4. Lee A, Chan S. Acupuncture and anaesthesia. Best Pract Res Clin Anaesthesiol. 2006;20:303–14.

5. Kawakita K, Okada K. Acupuncture therapy: Mechanism of action, efficacy, and safety: A potential intervention for psychogenic disorders? Biopsychosoc Med. 2014;8:4.

6. Lai HC, Lin YW, Hsieh CL. Acupuncture-Analgesia-Mediated Alleviation of Central Sensitization. Evid Based Complement Alternat Med. 2019 Mar 7;2019:6173412.

7. Kent ML,et.al.,The ACTTION-APS-AAPM Pain Taxonomy (AAAPT) Multidimensional Approach to Classifying Acute Pain Conditions.J Pain. 2017 May;18(5):479-489.

3. Medical indications for Acupuncture

In 1997 a landmark Consensus Statement on Acupuncture was issued by NIH, by a non-Federal, 12-member panel, representing the fields of acupuncture, pain, psychology, psychiatry, physical medicine and rehabilitation, drug abuse, family practice, internal medicine, health policy, epidemiology, statistics, physiology, biophysics, and the public.[1] Besides, 25 experts from these same fields presented data to the panel and a conference audience of 1,200. The objective of this NIH Consensus Statement was to inform the biomedical research and clinical practice communities of the results of the NIH Consensus Development Conference on Acupuncture. The statement provided information regarding the appropriate use of acupuncture and presented the conclusions and recommendations of the consensus panel regarding these issues. The literature was searched through Medline, and an extensive bibliography of references was provided to the panel and the conference audience. Experts prepared abstracts with relevant citations from the literature. Scientific evidence was given precedence over anecdotal clinical experience.

The conclusion of the panel was: while there have been many studies of its potential usefulness, many of these studies provide equivocal results because of design, sample size, and other factors. The issue is further complicated by inherent difficulties in the use of appropriate controls, such as placebos and sham acupuncture groups. However, promising results have emerged, for example, showing the efficacy of acupuncture in adult postoperative and chemotherapy nausea and vomiting and postoperative dental pain. There are other situations such as addiction, stroke rehabilitation, headache, menstrual cramps, tennis elbow, fibromyalgia, myofascial pain, osteoarthritis, low back pain, carpal tunnel syndrome, and asthma, in which acupuncture may be useful as an adjunct treatment or an acceptable alternative or be included in a comprehensive management program.[1] Further research is likely to uncover additional areas where acupuncture interventions will be useful.

On November 8–9, 2007, the Society for Acupuncture Research (SAR) hosted an international conference to mark the tenth anniversary of the landmark National Institutes of Health Consensus Development Conference on Acupuncture.[2,3] More than 300 acupuncture researchers, practitioners, students, funding agency personnel, and health policy analysts from 20 countries attended the SAR meeting held at the University of Maryland, School of Medicine, Baltimore, MD. Prominent invited speakers lectured in the area of clinical research. Specifically, included were: a review of German trials and observational studies on low-back pain (LBP), gonarthrosis, migraine, and tension-type headache (the Acupuncture Research Trials and the German Acupuncture Trials, plus observational studies). Also, it was considered a systematic review of acupuncture treatment for knee osteoarthritis (OA); and an overview of acupuncture trials in neurologic conditions, LBP, women's health, psychiatric disorders, and functional bowel disorders. A summary of the use of acupuncture in cancer care was also provided. Researchers involved in the German trials concluded that acupuncture is effective for treating chronic pain, but the correct selection of acupuncture points seems to play a limited role; no conclusions could be drawn about the placebo aspect of acupuncture, due to the design of the studies. Overall, when compared to sham, acupuncture did not show a benefit in treating knee OA or LBP, but acupuncture was better than a wait-list control and standard of care, respectively. In women's health, acupuncture is beneficial for patients with premenstrual syndrome, dysmenorrhea, several pregnancy-related conditions, and nausea in females who have cancers. Evidence on moxibustion for breech presentation, induction of labor, and reduction of menopausal symptoms is still inconclusive. In mental health, evidence for acupuncture's efficacy in treating neurologic and functional bowel disorder is still inconclusive. For chronic cancer-related problems such as pain, acupuncture may work well in stand-alone clinics; however, for acute or treatment-related symptoms, integration of acupuncture care into a busy and complex clinical environment is unlikely, unless compelling evidence of a considerable patient benefit can be established.

Several studies suggest that acupuncture-induced analgesia is mediated by the release of endogenous opioids. Results from human and animal studies, with the help of PET and fMRI, support these conclusions.

Although scientific evidence supports a physiological basis for acupuncture analgesia, the true efficacy of acupuncture for pain relief in humans remains in question, since both specific and non - specific factors may play a role in acupuncture therapy for pain, notably for orofacial pain. Many acupuncture trials have shown little or no superiority of correctly-performed (true) acupuncture over placebo/sham controls, in spite of the fact that both seem to be clinically effective. For example, research comparing acupuncture to sham acupuncture (placing a needle into a non- acupoint and just barely penetrating the skin) has shown that both treatments decreased the pain response to a pressure algometer applied to the masseter muscle in a group of myofascial pain patients.

Since 2007 many other pieces of evidence suggesting the usefulness of acupuncture in different medical fields were published.

Wang[4] suggests that acupuncture is a safe and effective therapy for managing cancer and treatment-related symptoms, such as nausea and vomiting and fatigue caused by chemotherapy.

In the treatment of Chronic Fatigue Syndrome, Combined Acupuncture and Moxibustion and Single Acupuncture and Moxibustion may have a better effect than other treatments. However, the included trials have relatively poor quality. Hence high-quality studies are needed to confirm the present findings.[5]

A growing interest in acupuncture is noticed in the US. Between 2002 and 2012, The number of acupuncture users and licensed acupuncturists increased by 50% and 100%, respectively, coinciding with increasing acknowledgment of the importance and efficacy of acupuncture over this time.[6]

A recent finding suggests that 90% of the benefits due to acupuncture sessions may last up to 12 months after the end of the treatment when compared to controls.[7]

A Cochrane review[8] suggests that acupuncture is likely to result in a decrease prostatitis symptoms and may not be associated with a higher incidence of adverse events.

There is low-quality evidence that real acupuncture has a moderate effect (approximate 12-point reduction on the 100-mm visual analogue scale) on musculoskeletal pain.[9]

MA might be efficacious in terms of pain relief and reduction of muscle irritability in myofascial pain syndrome patients, although additional well-designed/reported studies are required to determine the optimal number of sessions for the treatment of myofascial pain syndrome.[10]

Finally, acupuncture is included in the 2019 PDQ NIH Cancer Information Summaries, Health Professionals version.[11]

References

1. NIH Consensus Conference. Acupuncture. JAMA. 1998 Nov 4;280(17):1518-24. PDQ Integrative, Alternative, and Complementary Therapies Editorial Board.

2. Park J, Linde K, Manheimer E, Molsberger A, Sherman K, Smith C, Sung J, Vickers A, Schnyer R. The status and future of acupuncture clinical research. J Altern Complement Med. 2008 Sep;14(7):871-81.

3. Napadow V, Ahn A, Longhurst J, Lao L, Stener-Victorin E, Harris R, Langevin HM. The status and future of acupuncture mechanism research. J Altern Complement Med. 2008 Sep;14(7):861-9.

4. Wang G, Litscher G. Acupuncture for Neoplasms: An Update from the PubMed Database. Med Acupunct. 2015 Jun 1;27(3):151-157.

5. Wang T, Xu C, Pan K, Xiong H. Acupuncture and moxibustion for chronic fatigue syndrome in traditional Chinese medicine: a systematic review and meta-analysis. BMC Complement Altern Med. 2017 Mar 23;17(1):163

6. Cui J, Wang S, Ren J, Zhang J, Jing J. Use of acupuncture in the USA: changes over a decade (2002-2012). Acupunct Med. 2017 Jun;35(3):200-207.

7. MacPherson H, Vertosick EA, Foster NE, Lewith G, Linde K, Sherman KJ, Witt CM, Vickers AJ. The persistence of the effects of acupuncture after a course of treatment: a meta-analysis of patients with chronic pain. Pain. 2017 May;158(5):784-793.

8. Franco JVA, Turk T, Jung JH, Xiao YT, Iakhno S, Garrote V, Vietto V. Non-pharmacological interventions for treating chronic prostatitis/chronic pelvic pain syndrome: a Cochrane systematic review. BJU Int. 2018 Jul 18.

9. Yuan QL, Wang P, Liu L, Sun F, Cai YS, Wu WT, Ye ML, Ma JT, Xu BB, Zhang YG. Acupuncture for musculoskeletal pain: A meta-analysis and meta-regression of sham-controlled randomized clinical trials. Sci Rep. 2016 Jul 29;6:30675.

10. Wang R, Li X, Zhou S, Zhang X, Yang K, Li X. Manual acupuncture for myofascial pain syndrome: a systematic review and meta-analysis. Acupunct Med. 2017 Aug;35(4):241-250.

11. Acupuncture (PDQ®): Health Professional Version. 2019 Apr 19. PDQ Cancer Information Summaries [Internet]. Bethesda (MD): National Cancer Institute (US); 2002-. Available from http://www.ncbi.nlm.nih.gov/books/NBK65714/

4. Dry Needling, trigger point therapy and acupuncture

What is the difference between Dry Needling, trigger point therapy and acupuncture?

On the official website of the National Center for Complementary and Integrative Health of the U.S. National Institutes of Health, the definition of acupuncture has been expanded and described as a family of procedures involving the stimulation of points on the body using a variety of techniques. The acupuncture technique that has been most often studied scientifically involves penetrating the skin with thin, solid, metallic needles that are manipulated by the hands or by electrical stimulation. Acupuncture practitioners commonly use acupuncture needles that are solid, filiform metallic needles (although stone needles and bamboo needles were used in ancient times.) Practiced in China and other Asian countries for thousands of years, acupuncture is one of the key components of traditional Chinese medicine.

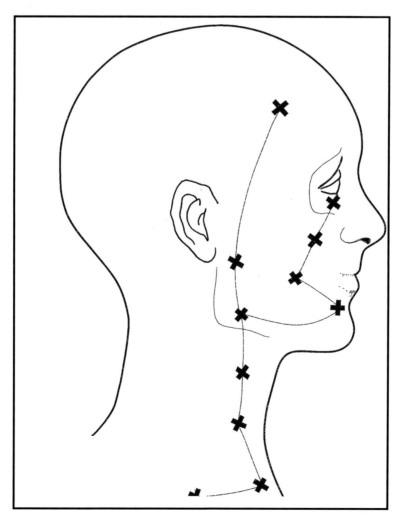

Western Trigger Point Therapy as popularized by Janet Travell, consisted of injecting local anesthetic into painful areas of muscles. In doing research, some investigators compared injecting local anesthetic into painful areas of muscles, to a control group of just needling the area without injecting any substance, and they found that both treatments were effective. That was the beginning of dry needling.[1]

Dry needling evolved from Trigger Point Therapy as popularized by Travell, at first using a hollow needle without local anesthetic to activate the trigger point. Acupuncture needles were not utilized for dry needling until 1979, when Acupuncture became popular in the United States. Acupuncture needles were safer and produced less bleeding and bruising.[2]

Melzack R, Et, Al, looked at 2 criteria: the spatial distribution and the associated pain pattern of trigger points and compared them to classical acupuncture points. A 71% correspondence was found, suggesting that Trigger points and acupuncture points, though discovered independently, represent the same phenomenon.

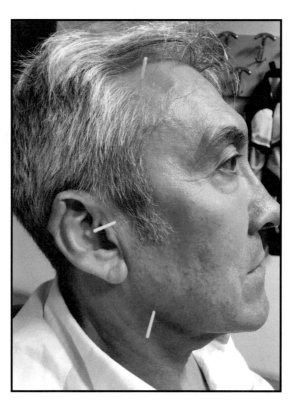

Dry needling and Trigger Point Therapy are both used to treat Myofascial pain, one of the temporomandibular disorders (TMD), which is a frequently encountered pain syndrome of muscle/connective tissue that is characterized by localized, hypersensitive spots in one or more palpable taut bands of skeletal muscle fiber, also known as myofascial trigger points.[4]

In traditional acupuncture, any active trigger point, anywhere on the body, is called an Ashi point, and those points are usually needled as part of the acupuncture treatment. In Dry Needling and Trigger Point therapy, only the Ashi points are needled. Therefore all trigger points would qualify as acupuncture points by being Ashi points. Acupuncture treats Myofascial pain by needling the Ashi points, which are identical to the trigger points. All three treatment modalities use the same points, the only difference is that acupuncture may add additional non Ashi points to provide generalized analgesia, calm anxiety and provide a feeling of well-being.

We found in our study of acupuncture for myofascial pain of the masticatory muscles that there was no difference statistically between treating pain with either verum acupuncture or sham acupuncture, and this evidence could indicate that even needling on a non-acupuncture point can have pain relief.[3]

In a blinded, placebo controlled RCT, 52 subjects got dry needling vs sham needling, and the results showed that dry needling appears to be an effective treatment method in relieving the pain and tenderness of myofascial trigger points.[4]

A study comparing deep or sham dry needling at the most painful point on the masseter muscle showed that dry needling into active TP's in the masseter induced significant increases in PPT levels and maximal jaw opening when compared to the sham.[5]

There have been several systematic reviews and meta-analysis of dry needling for myofascial pain of the masticatory and cervical muscles with positive results. In a review and meta-analysis of dry needling for myofascial trigger points, 20 RCT's involving 839 patients were reviewed for meta-analysis. The results suggested that dry needling relieved TP pain in neck and shoulders in the short and medium term.[6]

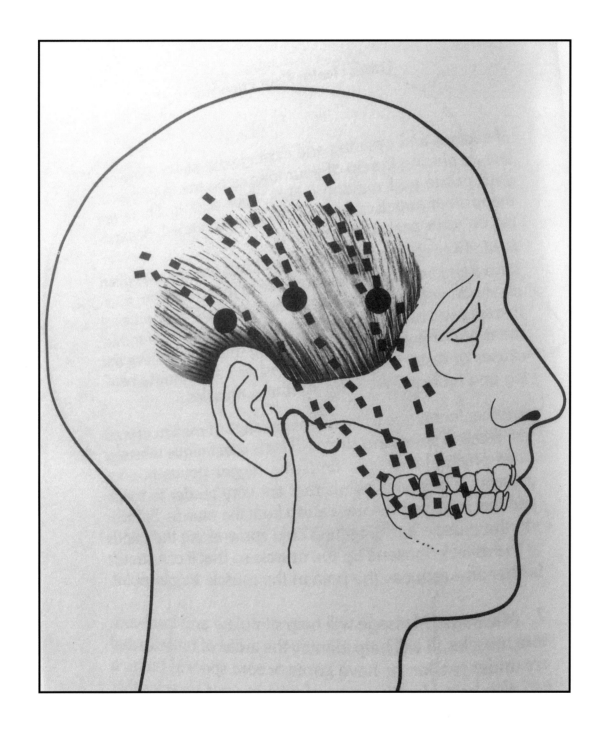

References

1. J Travell, SH Rinzler. The myofascial genesis of pain. Postgrad Med. 1952;11(5):425–41.

2. Melzack R, Stillwell D, Fox E., in their paper, Trigger points and acupuncture points for pain: correlations and implications, Pain. 1977 Feb;3(1):3-23

3. Goddard G, Karibe H, McNeill C, Villafuerte E, Acupuncture and sham acupuncture reduce muscle pain in myofascial pain patients,J Orofac Pain. 2002 Winter;16(1):71-6.

4. Dıraçoğlu D, et al, Effectiveness of dry needling for the treatment of temporomandibular myofascial pain: a double-blind, randomized, placebo controlled study,J Back Musculoskelet Rehabil. 2012;25(4):285-90.

5. Fernández-Carnero J, Short-term effects of dry needling of active myofascial trigger points in the masseter muscle in patients with temporomandibular disorders. J Orofac Pain. 2010 Winter;24(1):106-12

6. Liu. L, et al, Systematic Re4view and meta analysis of dry needling for myofascial trigger points, Arch Phys Med Rehabil. 2015 May;96(5):944-55

5. Laser Acupuncture

Laser Acupuncture

Acupuncture points can be activated by many different modalities. Needles are the most common, but acupressure, heat using Moxa, transcutaneous electrical nerve stimulation (TENS); and increasingly more popular, lasers, are also used.[1,2]

Laser acupuncture—the use of nonthermal, low-intensity laser irradiation to stimulate acupuncture points—has become more common among acupuncture practitioners in recent years. Laser acupuncture is promoted as a safer pain-free alternative to traditional acupuncture, with minimal adverse effects and greater efficacy. Laser Acupuncture, also termed low-level laser therapy, dates back to the 1970s with successful treatment of asthma and hypertension in the Soviet Union.[3]

Various lasers have been used, and there is no universally accepted laser or technique for Laser Acupuncture. In 1984 Zhou, using a beam from a 2.8-6 mW helium-neon laser apparatus that was delivered and focused to a red spot on the selected skin point of the patient, reported satisfactory results in an advanced clinical trial with laser acupuncture anesthesia for minor operations in the oro-maxillofacial region (610 cases (562 cases of difficult exodontia and 48 cases of various minor operations in the oro-maxillofacial region).[4]

In a human study, Laser Acupuncture of the acupoint BL 67, empirically associated with ophthalmic disorders, resulted in activation of visual cortex areas on fMRI. Sham acupuncture at that acupoint did not show activation. Laser Acupuncture has been shown to elicit cerebral activation, with involved brain areas corresponding to specific acupoints.[5]

Laser Acupuncture has also been incorporated into veterinary medicine as a way to accelerate healing in cases such as spinal-cord injury.[6]

Laser Acupuncture may be the preferred acupuncture modality for specific patient populations—such as geriatric and pediatric patients—because it is noninvasive, pain-free, and possibly associated with fewer adverse effects. The treatment length of an individual Laser Acupuncture session (10–60 seconds per acupuncture site) is shorter than that with metal needles (10–30-minute retention time), which can reduce the treatment time significantly.[7]

One clear difference between needle acupuncture and Laser Acupuncture is that Laser Acupuncture does not physically penetrate the skin. Despite greater understanding of Laser Acupuncture, it is unclear how nonthermal, low-intensity laser irradiation stimulates acupoints, and it is possible that the mechanism of Laser Acupuncture is entirely separate from our present understanding of acupuncture. Current theories postulate that low-level laser therapy could have a positive effect on modulating inflammation, pain, and tissue repair, given appropriate irradiation parameters.[8]

Portable Laser Acupuncture machines can offer convenient, efficient, and cost-effective treatment. Application of Laser Acupuncture involves many considerations, including existing data, technical parameters, clinical indications, safety, and future research to promote evidence-based clinical practices.[9]

Because the lasers used in Laser Acupuncture are Class 3b lasers, irradiation could potentially cause serious eye damage; therefore, patients and providers must wear protective eyewear during treatment. In addition, other precautions should be undertaken, including not directing the laser toward the fetus if a patient is pregnant, not irradiating the heart region of patients with cardiac conditions, and avoiding hemorrhagic areas and the gonads. The epiphyseal line in children should be avoided, and children younger than age 2 should not receive Laser Acupuncture. Direct irradiation of tumors should be avoided because it may stimulate their growth[10]

In 2008, Baxter and colleagues[11] conducted a systematic review of randomized controlled trials (RCTs) to examine the clinical effectiveness of Laser Acupuncture. These researchers identified moderate evidence supporting Laser Acupuncture as an effective treatment for reducing myofascial pain and moderate evidence supporting the use of Laser Acupuncture for postoperative nausea and vomiting. In 2015, Law and colleagues[12] conducted a systematic review and similarly reported moderate evidence supporting the use of Laser Acupuncture for managing musculoskeletal pain, when applied in appropriate treatment dosages.

Inflammation reduction comparable to that of nonsteroidal anti-inflammatory drugs has been reported with animal studies that used red and near-infrared LLLT, with laser outputs ranging from 2.5 to 100 mW and delivered energy doses ranging from 0.6 to 9.6 Joules. Human studies have shown similar anti-inflammatory effects with low-level laser therapy, which may account for many of the associated positive clinical effects.[13]

Lasers with output exceeding 500 mW, which are used for heating and direct tissue effects (e.g., tissue coagulation in surgery applications) are categorized as Class 4 "hard" lasers.[14] In contrast, lasers used for acupuncture applications typically have a power output of 5–499 mW and are categorized as Class 3b "soft" lasers. Some commercially available "laser devices" are not true lasers; rather, they use arrays of red or infrared light-emitting diodes (LEDs) that have noncollimated light outputs. Noncollimated light scatters and reflects at superficial skin layers, which limits energy penetration through the skin. Because the acupuncture meridians and their acupoints are thought to exist in the myofascial layer of the body,[15] the low energy penetration of LED devices theoretically fails to stimulate acupoints. However, LED devices often compensate for light scatter by using higher-output LEDs to enhance energy penetration through the skin.

The power density of a laser, defined as laser energy supplied per area (W/cm^2), influences its depth of energy penetration. A 50-mW laser with a beam size of $1 cm^2$ has an energy density of $0.05 W/cm^2$, whereas the same power laser with a beam size of $1 mm^2$ has an energy density of $5 W/cm^2$. A higher energy density results in deeper energy penetration through skin.

Energy transmission through the skin is also affected by absorption of light energy by skin structures. Light wavelengths from 650 to 900 nm have the best penetration through skin. Lower wavelengths are absorbed by melanin and hemoglobin, and wavelengths longer than 900 nm are absorbed by water. With a well-focused laser beam, red wavelengths (– 648 nm) can penetrate 2–4 cm beneath the skin surface, and infrared wavelengths (– 810 nm) can penetrate up to 6 cm. [16,17]

Laser Acupuncture devices may have 1 beam (a single-channel device) or multiple beams. The Weber* laser needle system [16] has 12 separate lasers to treat multiple acupoints simultaneously.

Low-level laser stimulation of acupoints has been reported to influence peripheral and central nervous system activity. In an animal study, stimulation of acupoints LI 4 and ST 36 with a 780-nm laser decreased somatosensory-evoked potentials activated by noxious stimulation of tooth pulp.[18] The reduction observed with lasers was similar to that associated with electro acupuncture of the same acupoints. The reduced amplitude of somatosensory-evoked potentials corresponded to the production of analgesia.

Conclusions

Laser Acupuncture is a promising approach to acupuncture that deserves attention, both for less morbidity and a similar efficacy. It is often used by medical and dental practioners, chiropractrs, and physical therapists that do not meet the governmental certification for practicing acupuncture. Using lasers to stimulate acupuncture points is often not considered to be acupuncture, which is defined as the insertion of needles in acupoints. Further studies are needed to increase our knowledge on the mechanisms of action, and efficacy of lasers; whether lasers are similar or different from traditional needling techniques.

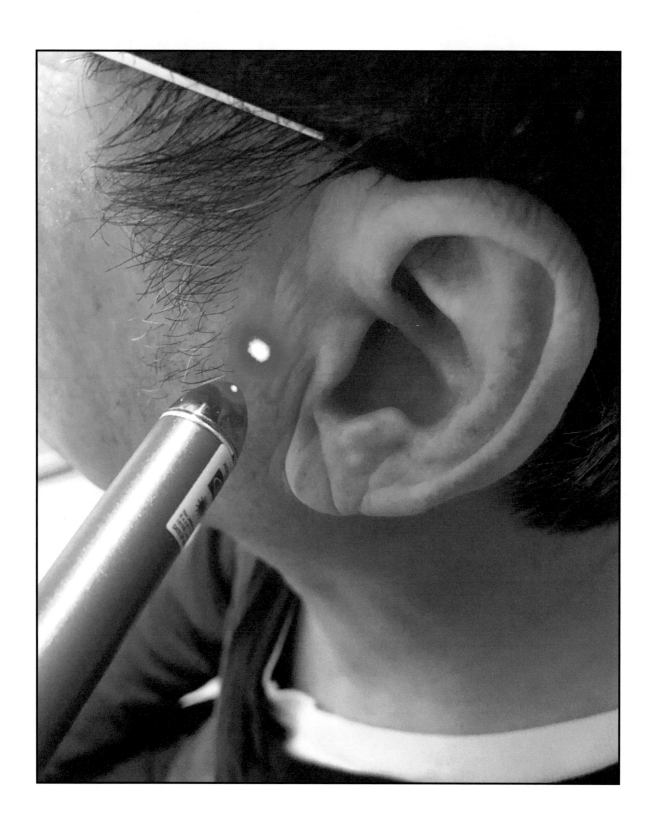

References

1. Chon TY, Lee MC. Acupuncture. Mayo Clin Proc. 2013; 88(10):1141–1146.

2. Chon TY, Mallory MJ, Yang J, Bublitz et al. Laser Acupuncture: A Concise Review. 2019:1343

3. Gamaleya NF. Laser biomedical research in the USSR. In: Wolbarsht ML, ed. Laser Applications in Medicine and Biology. New York: Plenum; 1977.

4. Zhou YC. An advanced clinical trial with laser acupuncturanesthesia for minor operations in the oro-maxillofacial region. Lasers Surg Med. 1984;4(3):297–303.

5. Siedentopf CM, Golaszewski SM, Mottaghy FM, Ruff CC, Felber S, Schlager A. Functional magnetic resonance imaging detects activation of the visual association cortex during laser acupuncture of the foot in humans. Neurosci Lett. 2002;327(1):53–56.

6. Riegel RJ, Godbold JCJ. Part 1: The history of laser therapy. In: Laser Therapy in Veterinary Medicine. Photobiomodulation, 1st ed: Hoboken, NJ: Wiley–Blackwell; 2017:3–6.

7. Hu WL, Chang CH, Hung YC, Tseng YJ, Hung IL, Hsu SF. Laser acupuncture therapy in patients with treatment-resistant temporomandibular disorders. PLoS One. 2014;9(10):e110528.

8. Chung H, Dai T, Sharma SK, Huang YY, Carroll JD, Hamblin MR. The nuts and bolts of low-level laser (light) therapy. Ann Biomed Eng. 2012;40(2):516–533.

9. Li C, Zhen H. Design of the laser acupuncture therapeutic instrument. Conf. Proc IEEE Eng Med Biol Soc. 2006;1:4107-10.

10. Uemoto L, Nascimento de Azevedo R, Almeida Alfaya T, Nunes Jardim Reis R, Depes de Gouveˆa CV, Cavalcanti Garcia MA. Myofascial trigger point therapy: Laser therapy and dry needling. Curr Pain Headache Rep. 2013;17(9):357.

11. Baxter GD, Bleakley C, McDonough S. Clinical effectiveness of laser acupuncture: A systematic review. J Acupunct Meridian Stud. 2008;1(2):65–82.

12. Law D, McDonough S, Bleakley C, Baxter GD, Tumilty S. Laser acupuncture for treating musculoskeletal pain: A sys- tematic review with meta-analysis. J Acupunct Meridian Stud. 2015;8(1):2–16.

13. Bjordal JM, Lopes-Martins RAB, Joensen J, Iversen VV. The anti-inflammatory mechanism of low level laser therapy and its relevance for clinical use in physiotherapy. Physical Ther Rev. 2010;15(4):286–293.

14. International Electrotechnical Commission (IEC). IEC 60825-1:2014/ISH1:2017 Interpretation Sheet 1—Safety of Laser Products—Part 1: Equipment Classification and Requirements. Geneva: International Electrotechnical Commission; 2017. Online document at: www.nen.nl/pdfpreview/preview_242393.pdf Accessed May 20, 2019.

15. O'Connor J, Bensky D. Acupuncture: A Comprehensive Text. Seattle: Eastland Press; 1981.

16. Weber M, Fussganger-May T, Wolf T. "Needles of Light": A new therapeutic approach. Med Acupunct. 2007;19(3):141–150.

17. Romberg H. How is (laser)-light working? COMED. 2001;11: 27–33.

18. Sing T, Yang MM. Electroacupuncture and laser stimulation treatment: Evaluated by somatosensory evoked potential in conscious rabbits. Am J Chin Med. 1997;25(3–4):263–271.

6. Acupuncture for Dentistry

A 2019 Pubmed search (keywords: acupuncture, dentistry, limit: reviews) retrieved 69 papers. From this search, some conclusions can be drawn.

In the Geneva WHO 2003 report, pain in dentistry (including dental pain, facial pain and postoperative pain, were listed among the conditions for which acupuncture has been proven to be successful through controlled trials, to be an effective treatment. There are numerous reports of randomized controlled trials on the analgesic effect of acupuncture for postoperative pain caused by various dental procedures.[1,2]

Some of the dental conditions for which acupuncture can be used effectively include:

- Dental pain, acute and postoperative

- Dental anxiety

- Nausea and gag reflex.

- Xerostomia (dry mouth) and sialorrrhea

- Paresthesia or anesthesia of the oral and perioral structures.

- Orofacial Pain (see next chapter)

Acupuncture for Pain

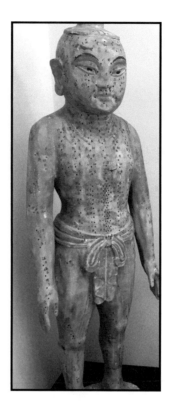

The results of this study indicate that acupuncture analgesia could be a technical adjunct to pain control in patients with acute dental pain, contributing to the restoration of health with social benefit.[3]

Pain by the injection, more than the obvious following numbness, is the fear that acupuncture mainly addresses in its action.[4]

Acupuncture cannot be administered by a non-trained clinician since it is not a risk-free practice. Nevertheless, the general population agrees with this approach and the popularity of acupuncture increases.[5]

References

1. Rosted P Introduction to acupuncture in dentistry. Br Dent J. 2000 Aug 12;189(3):136-40.

2. Naik PN, Kiran RA, Yalamanchal S, Kumar VA, Goli S, Vashist N. Acupuncture: An Alternative Therapy in Dentistry and Its Possible Applications. Med Acupunct. 2014 Dec 1;26(6):308-314.

3. Grillo CM, Wada RS, da Luz Rosário de Sousa M. Acupuncture in the management of acute dental pain. J Acupunct Meridian Stud. 2014 Apr;7(2):65-70

4. Armfield JM1, Milgrom P. A clinician guide to patients afraid of dental injections and numbness. SAAD Dig. 2011 Jan;27:33-9

5. Gupta D, Dalai DR, Swapnadeep, Mehta P, Indra BN, Rastogi S, Jain A, Chaturvedi M, Sharma S, Singh S, Gill S, Singh N, Gupta RK. Acupuncture (zhēn jiǔ) - an emerging adjunct in routine oral care. J Tradit Complement Med. 2014 Oct;4(4):218-23

Acupuncture for Gagging

Nausea, gagging, and the urge of vomit as seen in hyperparasympathetic subjects, are challenging situations in the dental setting when trying to make impressions, or to perform routine oral hygiene, or dental restorations. Generally, the studies on the efficacy of acupuncture science on controlling gag reflex are not vast enough to provide a reliable and comprehensive conclusion. However, based on published researches, the stimulation of acupuncture points, especially CV-24 and PC-6, seems to provide a remarkable reduction on gag reflex and it might be suggested for the practitioner to consider these points during gagging. Finally, two medical conditions; xerostomia (hyposalivation), and the opposite, sialorrhea (hypersalivation) can take advantage of an acupuncture approach, although present evidence is not sufficient to draw definitive conclusions.

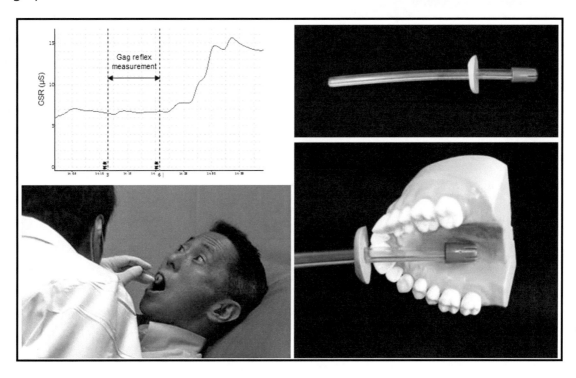

Technique for measuring gag reflex

The gag reflex is a normal, protective, physiological mechanism that occurs to prevent foreign objects and noxious material from entering the pharynx, larynx, and trachea.[1] A proportion of the population has a profound and exaggerated reflex that can cause acute limitation of a patient's ability to accept dental treatment and a clinician's ability to provide it.[2] A recent study reported that the prevalence of self-reported gagging during dental treatment was 8.2%.[3] Despite numerous management strategies, some patients cannot accept even simple dental treatment.

There are two different factors in the gag reflex. Somatic gagging is initiated by sensory nerve stimulation from direct contact; psychogenic gagging is modulated by higher centers in the brain.[4] In somatic gagging, touching a trigger area induces the reflex. Although trigger areas are specific to individuals, sites such as the lateral border of the tongue and certain parts of the palate commonly elicit the reflex.[5] Psychogenic gagging can be induced without direct contact; the sight, sound, smell or thought of dental treatment can induce the reflex.[4] A precise division between the somatic and psychogenic reflexes is not possible.[4] Thus, some patients who demonstrate a severe somatically induced gag reflex at the dentist are able to brush their teeth, eat, and place other objects in their own mouth without problems.[5]

Other factors, such as nasal obstruction, gastrointestinal disorders, heavy smoking, ill-fitting partial or full dentures, variation in the anatomy of the soft palate, and previous unpleasant experiences during dental treatment, may indirectly contribute to the exaggerated gag reflex.[5] suggested that Unpleasant dental experiences result in patients expecting to gag during future similar episodes. A previous study also reported that gagging was associated with female patients, increased dental anxiety, anxious depression, and neuroticism.[3]

A number of strategies have been used to control the profound gag reflex and allow dental care. They include relaxation, distraction, and desensitization techniques; psychological and behavioral therapies; local anesthesia, conscious sedation, and general anesthesia techniques; and complementary medicine therapies such as hypnosis, acupressure, and acupuncture. These strategies have been variably successful, but it may be necessary to try multiple methods to find the appropriate technique for an individual.

A clinical study assessed the role of acupuncture for treating orthodontic patients who experienced a gag reflex. The study investigated two acupuncture approaches for orthodontic patients with the gag reflex. Each patient had an upper dental alginate impression taken and that patient's gag reflex was evaluated using the Gagging Severity Index (GSI). After acupuncture was administered, a second impression was taken, and the Gagging Prevention Index (GPI) was used to evaluate the patient's gag reflex. A significant decrease in GPI values, compared to GSI values, was observed in the treatment groups, compared with a placebo group. The researchers concluded that acupuncture points used were effective in controlling the gag reflex in orthodontic patients.

Several points are introduced as acupuncturing points for various medical procedures. A review of literature found different acupuncturing points have been proposed for elimination of gagging. The PC-6 point has remarkable anti-gagging effects if stimulation is applied correctly. On the same acupuncture point, a study on 33 patients with severe gagging reflex who required alginate impression form maxillary arch. In that study, used visual analog scaling (VAS), gagging severity index (GSI) and gagging prevention index (GPI) were used for qualitative measurements. They stated no significant correlation between the patient's expectation and the actual reductions in gagging. Also, they indicated that PC-6 point was effective for controlling gagging reflex during preparing maxillary impression procedure. The PC-6 point was again observed. They examined the acupuncturing of that point for eliminating the induced gagging during stimulation of the soft palate and the sides of the tongue by medical wood sticks. Their results also supported the significant reduction of gag reflex.[5]

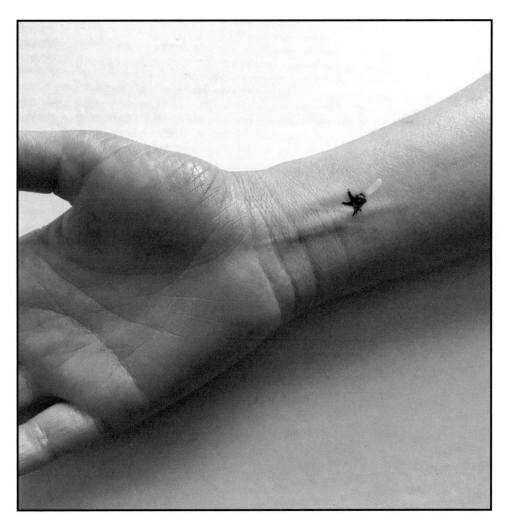

CONCLUSION

Generally, the studies on the efficacy of acupuncture on controlling gag reflex are not vast enough to provide a reliable and comprehensive conclusion. However, based on published researches, the stimulation of acupuncture points, especially CV-24 and PC-6, seems to provide a remarkable reduction on gag reflex and it might be suggested for practitioner to consider these points during gagging.

References

1. Bassi GS, Humphris GM, Longman LP. The etiology and management of gagging: A review of the literature. J Prosthet Dent. 2004;91:459–67. [PubMed]

2. Dickinson CM, Fiske J. A review of gagging problems in dentistry: 2. Clinical assessment and management. Dent Update. 2005;32:74. [PubMed]

3. Morrish RB. Method of Suppression and Prevention of the Gag Reflex. Google Patents. 2001

4. Hotta H. Case report of difficult dental prosthesis insertion due to severe gag reflex. Bull Tokyo Dent Coll. 2012;53:133–9. [PubMed]

5. Alireza Daneshkazemi, Pedram Daneshkazemi,[1] Amin Davoudi,[2] Hamid Badrian,[3] andVahid Pourtalebi Firouzabadi[4] Is acupuncturing effective in controlling the gag reflex during dental procedures? A review of literature, Anesth Essays Res. 2016 May-Aug; 10(2): 173–177.

Acupuncture for Dental Anxiety

Acupuncture has been used to manage dental anxiety.[1] In 2010, Rosted et al.[2] examined the effect of acupuncture administered prior to dental treatment on patients' level of anxiety. Eight dentists submitted 21 case reports regarding their treatments for dental anxiety. Anxiety levels were assessed by the Beck Anxiety Inventory (BAI). BAI score was assessed before and after acupuncture treatment. All patients received an acupuncture treatment for 5 minutes prior to the planned dental treatment. There was a significant reduction in median value of BAI scores after treatment with acupuncture (26.5 reduced to 11.5; $P<0.01$), and it was possible to perform the planned dental treatment in all 20 cases after acupuncture treatment.

References

1. Appukuttan DP Strategies to manage patients with dental anxiety and dental phobia: literature review. Clin Cosmet Investig Dent. 2016 Mar 10;8:35-50

2. Rosted P, Bundgaard M, Gordon S, Pedersen AM.,Acupuncture in the management of anxiety related to dental treatment: a case series., Acupunct Med. 2010 Mar;28(1):3-5.

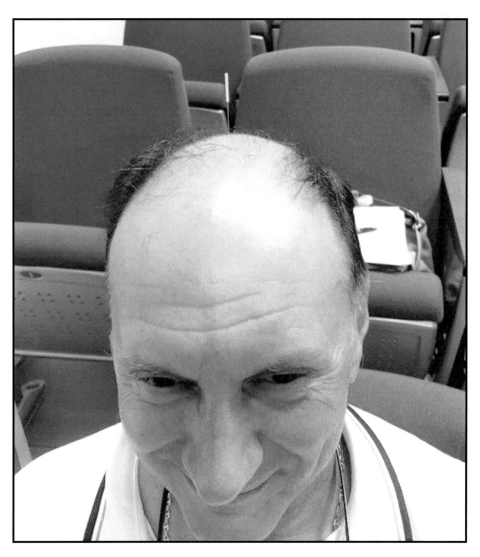

7. Acupuncture for Orofacial Pain

Orofacial pain (OFP) is a general term covering any pain which is felt in the mouth, jaws and the face. Orofacial pain is a common symptom, and there are many causes. It is estimated that over 95% of cases of orofacial pain result from dental causes. After dental pain, the second most common cause of orofacial pain are the Temporomandibular Disorders (TMD). All other causes of orofacial pain are rare in comparison, although the full differential diagnosis is extensive. [1]

The term **Temporomandibular Disorders (TMD)** comprise a number of conditions characterized by signs and symptoms involving the temporomandibular joint (TMJ), masticatory muscles, or both. [2]

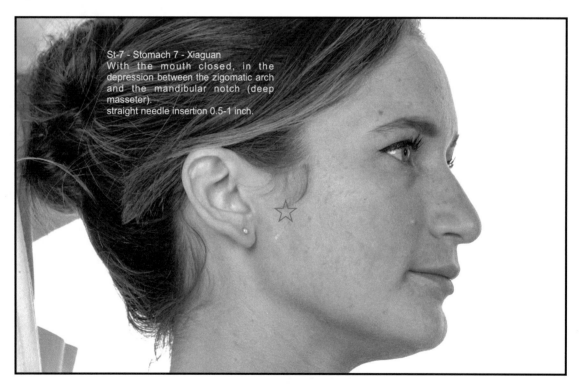

St-7 - Stomach 7 - Xiaguan
With the mouth closed, in the depression between the zigomatic arch and the mandibular notch (deep masseter).
straight needle insertion 0.5-1 inch.

Acupuncture for temporomandibular disorders

Temporomandibular disorders (TMJ arthritis, TMJ synovitis, myofascial pain), TMD myalgia

Temporomandibular Disorders (TMD), (M26-60 to M26-63 according to ICD) are the second most common musculoskeletal conditions (after chronic low back pain) resulting in pain and disability.

General Considerations

Temporomandibular disorders (TMDs) are a set of musculoskeletal disorders affecting the temporomandibular joint (TMJ), the masticatory muscles, or both. Myofascial pain is characterized by localized, hypersensitive spots in palpable taut bands of muscle fibers (myofascial trigger points). These trigger points may be due to muscle overload from trauma or repetitive activities that cause abnormal stress on specific muscle groups. Clinically, patients complain of tenderness, headaches, restricted movement, and muscle stiffness and weakness.[1,2]

TMDs comprise many diverse diagnoses with similar signs and symptoms affecting the masticatory system, which can be acute, recurrent, or chronic. TMDs are rarely life threatening, but can impact heavily on an individual's quality of life. Studies show that about 3–7% of the population need tr TMDs comprise many diverse diagnoses with similar signs and symptoms affecting the masticatory system, which can be acute, recurrent, or chronic. TMDs are rarely life threatening, but can impact heavily on an individual's quality of life. Studies show that about 3–7% of the population need treatment.

TMDs occur disproportionately in women of childbearing age in a ratio of 4:1 to 6:1, and the role of estrogens seems to show an association. The prevalence drops off dramatically for both men and women after age 55.[3-5]

The cause of TMD is variable and uncertain, and it is thought to be multifactorial in most cases. Genetic factors have recently been implicated [6,7]. Most factors are not proven causal factors, but they are associated with TMDs. Predisposing factors increase the risk of TMDs (structural, metabolic, genetic and psychological conditions). Initiating (Precipitating) factors are trauma, both direct (eg, blows to the jaw), indirect (eg, whiplash injuries) or repetitive adverse loading like micro trauma, and sometimes stress. Micro trauma is caused by clenching and grinding of the teeth. Stress can also be a predisposing factor owing to the disruption of restorative sleep and the increase of nocturnal bruxism.

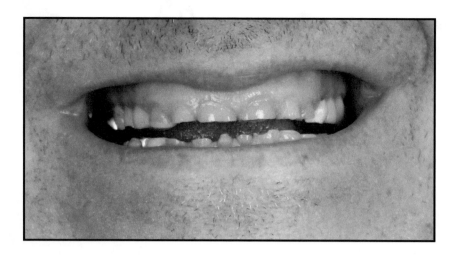

Perpetuating (Aggravating) factors that sustain a TMD are stress again, poor coping skills, persistent harmful habits such as clenching and grinding, and poor posture. Nonrestorative sleep also may be a major factor in the perpetuation of chronic jaw pain.[8-10]

Acupuncture is an increasingly utilized treatment option for myofascial pain in the United States. According to the 2007 National Health Interview Survey (NHIS), which included a comprehensive survey of complementary and alternative medicine use by Americans, an estimated 3.1 million adults and 150,000 children had used acupuncture in the previous year. Between the 2002 and 2007 NHIS, acupuncture use among adults increased by 0.3% (approximately 1 million people). In 1996, the United States Federal Drug Agency also promoted acupuncture needles from the investigational and experimental medical device category to the regular medical-device category, and the following year the National Institutes of Health (NIH) consensus statement on acupuncture supported the treatment efficacy of acupuncture for conditions such as pain and nausea.[3] Despite this increased recognition of acupuncture as a treatment for pain, much evidence for its effectiveness comes from poorly designed studies with inadequate controls and blinding procedures.

A variety of mechanisms have been proposed to explain the analgesic effects of acupuncture. These mechanisms are based on concepts that range from traditional views that center on imbalances of energy flow (chi) through the body, to modern Western views that stress the role of activated neural[14-17] and endogenous opioid systems.[18] The involvement of classic analgesic systems has been supported by neuroimaging and other studies performed on human and animal subjects.[19-22] It is also likely, however, that acupuncture involves a strong placebo component.[23,24] For example, while manual needle manipulation and electro acupuncture at the Hegu large intestine 4 (LI4) acupoint produced prominent decreases of blood oxygen level dependent signals (BOLD) in the posterior cingulate, superior temporal gyrus, and putamen/insula, so did sham acupuncture.[25] As more is learnt about the physiological basis of placebo analgesia,[26] it becomes increasingly important that its effects be separated from true, treatment-specific effects.

A systematic review of acupuncture for temporomandibular disorders found that there was moderate evidence that acupuncture is an effective intervention to reduce the symptoms associated with temporomandibular disorders.

Acupuncture for the treatment MYOFASCIAL PAIN

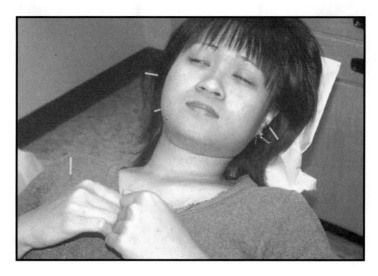

Increasing evidence supports the use of acupuncture in treating chronic conditions such as myofascial pain disorder. Myofascial pain is characterized by localized, hypersensitive spots in palpable taut bands of muscle fibers (myofascial trigger points). These trigger points may be due to muscle overload from trauma or repetitive activities that cause abnormal stress on specific muscle groups. Clinically, patients complain of tenderness, headaches, restricted movement, and muscle stiffness and weakness.[1,2]

Acupuncture is an increasingly utilized treatment option for myofascial pain in the United States. According to the 2007 National Health Interview Survey (NHIS), which included a comprehensive survey of complementary and alternative medicine use by Americans, an estimated 3.1 million adults and 150,000 children had used acupuncture in the previous year. Between the 2002 and 2007 NHIS, acupuncture use among adults increased by 0.3% (approximately 1 million people). In 1996, the United States Federal Drug Agency also promoted acupuncture needles from the investigational and experimental medical device category to the regular medical-device category, and the following year the National Institutes of Health (NIH) consensus statement on acupuncture supported the treatment efficacy of acupuncture for conditions such as pain and nausea.[3] Despite this increased recognition of acupuncture as a treatment for pain, much evidence for its effectiveness comes from poorly designed studies with inadequate controls and blinding procedures.

A variety of mechanisms have been proposed to explain the analgesic effects of acupuncture. These mechanisms are based on concepts that range from traditional views that center on imbalances of energy flow (chi) through the body, to modern Western views that stress the role of activated neural[14–17] and endogenous opioid systems.[18] The involvement of classic analgesic systems has been supported by neuroimaging and other studies performed on human and animal subjects.[19–22] It is also likely, however, that acupuncture involves a strong placebo component.[23,24]

Acupuncture is an increasingly utilized treatment option for myofascial pain in the United States. According to the 2007 National Health Interview Survey (NHIS), which included a comprehensive survey of complementary and alternative medicine use by Americans, an estimated 3.1 million adults and 150,000 children had used acupuncture in the previous year. Between the 2002 and 2007 NHIS, acupuncture use among adults increased by 0.3% (approximately 1 million people). In 1996, the United States Federal Drug Agency also promoted acupuncture needles from the investigational and experimental medical device category to the regular medical-device category, and the following year the National Institutes of Health (NIH) consensus statement on acupuncture supported the treatment efficacy of acupuncture for conditions such as pain and nausea.[3] Despite this increased recognition of acupuncture as a treatment for pain, much evidence for its effectiveness comes from poorly designed studies with inadequate controls and blinding procedures.

A variety of mechanisms have been proposed to explain the analgesic effects of acupuncture. These mechanisms are based on concepts that range from traditional views that center on imbalances of energy flow (chi) through the body, to modern Western views that stress the role of activated neural[14-17] and endogenous opioid systems.[18] The involvement of classic analgesic systems has been supported by neuroimaging and other studies performed on human and animal subjects.[19-22] It is also likely, however, that acupuncture involves a strong placebo component.[23,24]

Increasing evidence supports the use of acupuncture in treating chronic conditions such as myofascial pain disorder. A systematic review of, thirty-three trials with 1,692 patients, that used acupuncture for myofascial pain disorder found that the existing evidence suggests that most acupuncture therapies, including acupuncture combined with other therapies, are effective in decreasing pain and in improving physical function.

Smith et al tested 27 temporomandibular disorder myofascial pain subjects with six treatment sessions at two acupoints with real acupuncture or sham acupuncture using the Park Sham Device[37] and found a significant improvement in signs and symptoms of myofascial pain with real acupuncture but not with sham acupuncture.[38]

In a study with chronic myofascial pain of the jaw muscles. Participants were more likely to experience clinically significant reductions of jaw/face pain, jaw/face tightness, and neck pain with one treatment session at one acupoint of real versus sham acupuncture (75% versus 33% positive response rate of at least 30% pain reduction). Overall, the findings suggest that acupuncture has short-term beneficial clinical effects above general placebo analgesia induced from sham acupuncture for alleviating most myofascial pain symptoms.[39]

References

1. Simons DG, Travell JG, Simons PT. Upper Half of Body. 2. Vol. 1. Baltimore: Williams and Wilkins; 1999. Travell and Simons' Myofascial Pain and Dysfunction. The Trigger Point Manual.

2. Travell JG, Simons DG. Myofascial Pain and Dysfunction: The Trigger Point Manual. Vol. 1. Baltimore: Williams and Wilkins; 1983.

3. National Institutes of Health Consensus Panel. Acupuncture: National Institutes of Health Consensus Development Conference Statement. [Accessed June 22, 2007].http://consensus.nih.gov/t99y/1997acupuncture107html.htm.

4. Lytle CD. History of the Food and Drug Administration's regulation of acupuncture devices. J Altern Complement Med. 1996;2:253–256. [PubMed]

5. NIH Consensus Statement. Acupuncture. JAMA. 1998;280:1518–1524. [PubMed]

6. Audette J, Blinder RA. Acupuncture in the management of myofascial pain and headache. Curr Pain Headache Rep. 2003;7:395–401. [PubMed]

7. Harris RE, Clauw DJ. The use of complementary medical therapies in the management of myofascial pain disorders. Curr Pain Headache Rep. 2002;6:370–374. [PubMed]

8. Edelist G, Gross AE, Langer F. Treatment of low back pain with acupuncture. Can J Anaesth Soc. 1976;23:303–306. [PubMed]

9. Brandwein A, Corcos J. Extraction of incisors under acupuncture anesthesia: A standardized method. Am J Acup. 1975;3:352–354.

10. Goddard G, Karibe H, McNeil C, Villafuerte E. Acupuncture and sham acupuncture reduce muscle pain in myofascial pain patients. J Orofac Pain. 2002;16:71–76. [PubMed]

11. Kerr NW. Acupuncture for therapy and analgesia. A possible application in dental surgery. Br Dent J. 1973;134:201–204. [PubMed]

12. Lao L, Bergman S, Hamilton GR, Langenberg P, Herman B. Evaluation of acupuncture for pain control after oral surgery: A placebo-controlled trial. Arch Otolaryngol Head Neck Surg. 1999;125:567–572.[PubMed]

13. Lee MHM, Teng P, Zaretzky HH, Rubin M. Acupuncture anesthesia in dentistry. A clinical investigation. N Y State D J. 1973;39:299–301. [PubMed]

14. Mann F. Acupuncture analgesia in dentistry. Lancet. 1972;1:898–899. [PubMed]

15. Rosted P. The use of acupuncture in dentistry: A review. Compl Med Int. 1996;3:18–21.

16. Silva SA. Acupuncture for the relief of pain of facial and dental origin. Anesth Prog. 1989;36:244–245.[PMC free article] [PubMed]

17. Tany M, Matsudaira K, Sawatsugawa S, Manaka Y. Acupuncture analgesia and its application in dental practice. Am J Acup. 1974;2:287–295.

18. Shen J. Research on the neurophysiologies mechanisms of acupuncture: Review of selected studies and methodological issues. J Altern Complement Med. 2001;7(suppl 1):S121–S127. [PubMed]

19. Biella G, Sotgiu ML, Pellegata G, Paulesu E, Castiglioni I, Fazio F. Acupuncture produces central activations in pain regions. Neuroimage. 2001;14:60–66. [PubMed]

20. Bowsher D. Mechanisms of acupuncture. In: Filshie J, White A, editors. Medical Acupuncture: A Western Scientific Approach. London: Churchill Livingston; 1998. pp. 69–82.

21. Han JS. Neurochemical basis of acupuncture. Annu Rev Pharmacol Toxicol. 1982;22:193–220.[PubMed]

22. Hess J, Magelvang B, Simonsen H. Acupuncture versus metoprolol in migraine prophylaxis: A randomized trial of trigger point inacrivation. J Intern Med. 1994;235:451–456. [PubMed]

23. Ekblom A, Hansson P, Thomsson M, Thomas M. Increased post operative pain and consumption of analgesics following acupuncture. Pain. 1991;44:241–247. [PubMed]

24. Grabow L. Controlled study of the analgesic effectivity of acupuncture. Arzneimirtelforschung. 1994;44:554–558. [PubMed]

25. Kong J, Ma L, Gollub RL, et al. A pilot study of functional magnetic resonance imaging of the brain during manual and electroacupuncture stimulation of acupuncture point (LI-4 Hegu) in normal subjects reveals differential brain activation between methods. J Altern Complement Med. 2002;8:411–419.[PubMed]

26. Kaptchuk TJ. Acupuncture: Theory, efficacy, and practice. Ann Intern Med. 2002;137:702–703.

27. Shen Y, Goddard G. Short term effects of acupuncture on myofascial pain patients after clenching. Pain Pract. 2007;7:256–264. [PubMed]

28. Okeson JP. Management of Temporomandibular Disorders and Occlusion. 5. St. Louis: Mosby; 2003. pp. 339–342.

29. Stacher G, Wancura I, Bauer P, Lahoda R, Schulze D. Effect of acupuncture on pain threshold and pain tolerance determined by electrical stimulation of the skin: A controlled study. Am J Chin Med. 1975;3:143–149. [PubMed]

30. Hui KK, Liu J, Makris N, et al. Acupuncture modulates the limbic system and subcortical gray structures of the human brain: Evidence from fMRI studies in normal subjects. Hum Brain Mapp. 2000;9:13–25. [PubMed]

31. Tillu A, Roberts C, Tillu S. Unilateral versus bilateral acupuncture on knee function in advanced osteoarthritis of the knee: A prospective randomised trial. Acupunct Med. 2001;19:15–18. [PubMed]

32. Audette JF, Wang F, Smith H. Bilateral activation of motor unit potentials with unilateral needle stimulation of active moyfascial trigger points. Am J Phys Med Rehabil. 2004;83:368–374. [PubMed]

33. Goddard G, Shen Y, Steele B. A controlled trial of placebo vs real acupuncture. Pain. 2005;4:237–242.[PubMed]

34. Streitberger K, Kleinhenz J. Introducing a placebo needle into acupuncture research. Lancet. 1998;352:364–365. [PubMed]

35. Farrar JT, Young JP, Jr, LaMoreaux L, Werth JL, Poole RM. Clinical importance of changes in chronic pain intensity measured on an 11-point numerical pain rating scale. Pain. 2001;94:149–158. [PubMed]

36. Kam E, Eslick G, Campbell I. An audit of the effectiveness of acupuncture on musculoskeletal pain in primary health care. Acupunct Med. 2002;20:35–38. [PubMed]

37. Park J, White A, Stevinson C, Ernst E, James M. Validating a new non-penetrating sham acupuncture device: Two randomised controlled trials. Acupunct Med. 2002;20:168–174. [PubMed]

38. Smith P, Mosscrop D, Davies S, Sloan P, Al-Ani Z. The efficacy of acupuncture in the treatment of temporomandibular joint myofascial pain: A randomised controlled trial. J Dent. 2007;35:259–267.[PubMed]

39. Shen Y, Younger J, Goddard G, Mackey S, RCT of acupuncture for MFP of the jaw muscles, Orofac Pain. 2009 Fall;23(4):353-9.

Acupuncture for tension type headache TTHA

Tension type headache, the most common type of primary headaches, affects approximately 80% of the population. Mainly because of its high prevalence, the socio-economic consequences of tension type headache are significant.

The pain in tension type headache is usually bilateral, mild to moderate, is of a pressing or tightening quality, and is not accompanied by other symptoms. These patients often have very tender trigger points or Ashi points in their masticatory and cervical muscles that often refer pain and/or duplicate their headache.

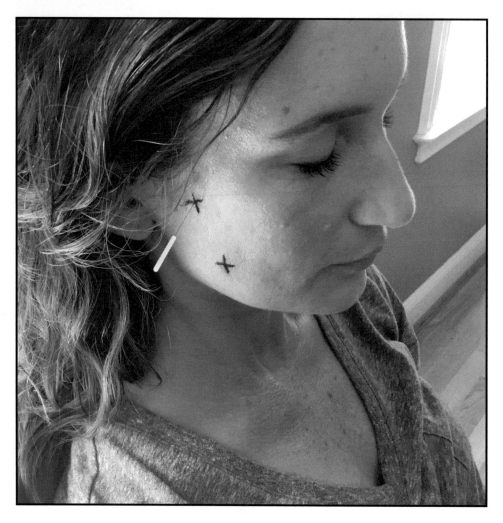

Patients with frequent or daily occurrence of tension type headache may experience significant distress because of the condition. The two main therapeutic avenues of tension type headache are acute and prophylactic treatment. Simple or combined analgesics are the mainstay of acute treatment. Prophylactic treatment is needed in case of attacks that are frequent and/ or difficult to treat. The first drugs of choice as preventatives of tension type headache are tricyclic antidepressants, with a special focus on amitriptyline, the efficacy of which having been documented in multiple double-blind, placebo-controlled studies. Among other antidepressants, the efficacy of mirtazapine and venlafaxine has been documented. There is weaker evidence about the efficacy of gabapentin, topiramate, and tizanidine.

Non-pharmacological prophylactic methods of tension type headache with a documented efficacy include certain types of psychotherapy and acupuncture.

Linde K, et al., in a recent Cochrane systematic review of Acupuncture for the prevention of tension-type headache looked at 12 trials with 2349 participants, concluded that the available evidence suggest that acupuncture is effective for treating frequent episodic or chronic tension-type headaches.

Acupuncture for Migraine Headaches

Migraine headache is characterized by a pre-headache phase that starts about 30 minutes before the actual headache. During this phase there often are visual symptoms ranging from blurriness to partial blindness. Other symptoms may be weakness, dizziness, mental confusion, or even tingling of the feet. These symptoms of Aura usually diminish within 30 minutes and the headache begins, usually on one side. Many people have Migraine headache without the aura or visual disturbances.

Migraine occurs in around 15% of adults and is ranked as the seventh most disabling disease amongst all diseases globally. Despite the available treatments many people suffer prolonged and frequent attacks which have a major impact on their quality of life. Chronic migraine is defined as 15 or more days of headache per month, at least eight of those days being migraine. People with episodic migraine have fewer than 15 headache days per month.

Acupuncture is often used for migraine prevention, and a systematic Cochrane review of 22 trials involving almost 5000 patients found that the available evidence suggests that adding acupuncture to symptomatic treatment of attacks reduces the frequency of headaches. Contrary to the previous findings, the updated evidence also suggests that there is an effect over sham, but this effect is small. The available trials also suggest that acupuncture may be at least similarly effective as treatment with prophylactic drugs. Acupuncture can be considered a treatment option for patients willing to undergo this treatment.

Acupuncture for the prevention of episodic migraine.

Linde, et al., in a 24-week randomized clinical trial (4 weeks of treatment followed by 20 weeks of follow-up), was undertaken to look at the long-term effects of true acupuncture compared with sham acupuncture and being placed in a waiting-list control group for migraine prophylaxis. Among patients with migraine without aura, true acupuncture may be associated with long-term reduction in migraine recurrence compared with sham acupuncture or assigned to a waiting list.

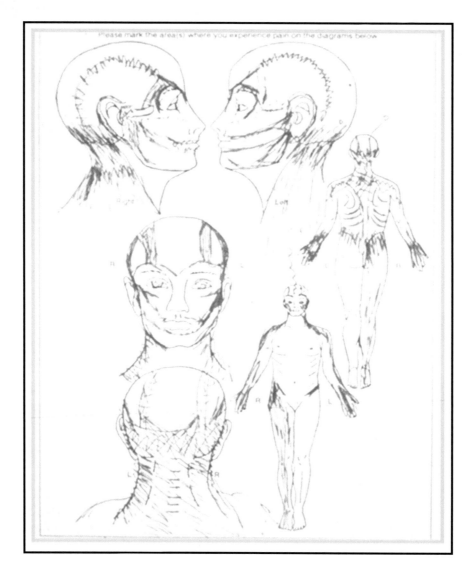

Acupuncture for Fibromyalgia

Fibromyalgia is a disorder characterized by widespread musculoskeletal pain concurrent with masticatory muscle pain. Fibromyalgia is often accompanied by fatigue and sleep disturbances., It involves pain for at least 3 months that involves both sides of the body, above and below the waist, as well as the axial skeleton. Researchers believe that fibromyalgia involves abnormal processing of peripheral stimuli within the central nervous system. Patients often suffer from fatigue; in fact fibromyalgia was once called chronic fatigue syndrome. Sleep is often disrupted by pain, and people often awaken tired, even though they report sleeping for long periods of time. Many of these people were previously high functioning; but their fibromyalgia impairs their ability to focus, pay attention and concentrate on mental tasks.

Women are more likely to develop fibromyalgia than are men. Many people who have fibromyalgia also have tension headaches, temporomandibular joint (TMJ) disorders, irritable bowel syndrome, anxiety and depression. In our clinic, we found that about 20% of the patients reporting with temporomandibular disorders actually had Fibromyalgia.

While there is no cure for fibromyalgia, a variety of medications can help control symptoms. Acupuncture, exercise, relaxation and stress-reduction measures also may help.[1]

A Cochrane Database Systematic Review looked at 9 trials with 395 participants, and concluded that there is low to moderate-level evidence that compared with no treatment and standard therapy, acupuncture improves pain and stiffness in people with fibromyalgia.

Acupuncture has been used with good success in the treatment of fibromyalgia. Vas, et al., in a randomized controlled multicenter trial of Acupuncture for fibromyalgia in primary care, blinded to participants and to data analysts was conducted in three primary care centers in southern Spain. A total of 153 participants completed the study. The study concluded that individualized acupuncture treatment in primary care in patients with fibromyalgia proved efficacious in terms of pain relief, compared with placebo treatment, and is recommended. The effect persisted at 1 year, and its side effects were mild and infrequent.[2]

References

1. https://www.nchmd.org/education/mayo-health-library/details/CON-20209450

2. Vas J et al, Acupuncture for fibromyalgia in primary care: a randomised controlled trial, Acupunct Med. 2016 Aug;34(4):257-66. doi: 10.1136/acupmed-2015-010950. Epub 2016 Feb 15

Acupuncture Treatment for Burning Mouth Syndrome

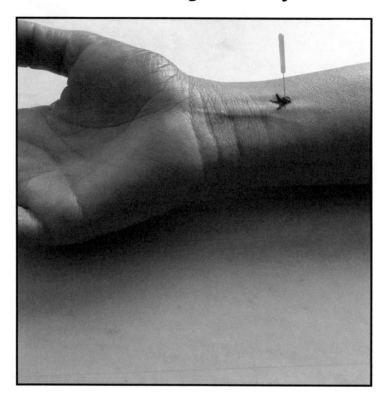

According to the International Headache Society Committee, Burning Mouth Syndrome (BMS) is an idiopathic condition consisting of an intraoral burning or dysesthetic sensation, recurring daily for more than 2 hours per day over more than 3 months, without clinically evident causative[1].

Prevalence of BMS increases with age in both males and females, but mainly affects females in the fifth to seventh decade. [2-4] BMS typically is a chronic problem of older adults, and more common in women than men, the female/male ratio of occurrence being 7:1, [2-8] and this population is prone to side effects from medication. BMS can involve multiple sites, but the tip of the tongue is the most common location (71%), followed by lips (50%), lateral border of tongue, (46%) and palate (46%). [9]

A systematic review of acupuncture or acupoint injection for management of burning mouth syndrome showed positive outcomes for the use of acupuncture therapy for BMS patients. [10]

A randomized controlled trial found that acupuncture and clonazepam are similarly effective for patients with BMS. [11] Another study found that combined acupuncture/auriculotherapy was effective in reducing the intensity of burning and improving quality of life. [12]

Koszewicz M, et al showed similar characteristics of autonomic nervous system disorders in burning mouth syndrome and Parkinson disease. Acupuncture could activate the autonomic response with changes in the sympathetic and parasympathetic nervous systems. Acupuncture has been shown to increase oral microcirculation in healthy volunteers, so it could influence oral microcirculation, resulting in a significant variation of the vascular pattern to which is associated a significant reduction of the burning sensation.

TREATMENT:

Our treatment protocol is for patients to receive the following acupuncture points: ear Shen Men, P6, and Ren 24.

Millennia stainless steel needles, size 40, 0.5 inch, for the ear points, and size 34, 1.5 inch, for the body points are inserted until a Chi reaction is elicited. The needles are left in place for 30 minutes

Results are usually positive with 3 weekly treatments, but some patients may need longer treatment.

Our published case series showed positive results.

We treated a series of eleven patients, 5 males and 6 females, ranging from 56 to 83 years of age, which were diagnosed with BMS, and were being actively treated with Klonopin. Acupuncture treatments were administered weekly for five weeks. At the first, third and fifth weekly session, their pain and restfulness visual analog scales (VAS) were recorded before the acupuncture. All adverse events were recorded.

The ratings for pain and rest were significantly reduced during 3-time treatment periods (pain, $P = 0.001$; rest, $P = 0.001$. There were no adverse events. These results give us additional confidence in our treatment protocols.

References:

1. The International Classification of Headache Disorders, Headache Classification Committee of the International Headache Society (IHS). Cephalalgia 2013; 33:629-808.

2. Jaaskelainen S, Woda A. Burning mouth syndrome. Cephalalgia 2017; 37:627–47.

3. Coculescu E, Tovaru S, Coculescu B. Epidemiological and etiological aspects of burning mouth syndrome. J Med Life. 2014 Sep 15; 7(3):305-9

4. Dahiya P, Kamal R, Kumar M, Niti, Gupta R, Chaudhary K. Burning mouth syndrome and menopause. Int J Prev Med 2013; 4:15-20.

5. Ferguson MM, Carter J, Boyle P, Hart DM, Lindsay R. Oral complaints related to climacteric symptoms in oophorectomized women. J R Soc Med 1981; 74:492–8.

6. Ship JA, Grushka M, Lipton JA, Mott AE, Sessle BJ, Dionne RA. Burning mouth syndrome: An update. J Am Dent Assoc 1995; 126:842-53.

7. Grushka M. Clinical features of burning mouth syndrome. Oral Surg Oral Med Oral Pathol 1987; 63:30–6.

8. Van Der Waal I. The burning mouth syndrome. Copenhagen: Munskgaard, 1990: 5-90.

9. Miyamoto S, Ziccardi VB. Burning Mouth syndrome. Mt Sinai J Med 1998; 65:343-7.

10. Yan Z1, Ding N, Hua H, A systematic review of acupuncture or acupoint injection for management of burning mouth syndrome, Quintessence Int. 2012 Sep;43(8):695-701.

11. Kvesic A, Zavoreo I, Basic Kes V, Vucicevic Boras V, Ciliga D, Gabric D, Vrdoljak D, The effectiveness of acupuncture versus clonazepam in patients with burning mouth syndrome, Acupunct Med. 2015 Aug;33(4):289-92.

12. Franco FR1, Castro LA2, Borsatto MC3, Silveira EA4, Ribeiro-Rotta RF1,Combined Acupuncture and Auriculotherapy in Burning Mouth Syndrome Treatment: A Preliminary Single-Arm Clinical Trial, J Altern Complement Med. 2017 Feb;23(2):126-134.

Acupuncture for Trigeminal Neuralgia

Trigeminal neuralgia is a chronic pain condition that affects the trigeminal nerve, which carries sensation from the face to the brain. With trigeminal neuralgia, even mild stimulation of your face, such as from brushing your teeth or putting on makeupmay trigger a jolt of excruciating pain.

Typically, trigeminal neuralgia is characterized by episodes of severe electric-like pain that lasts for seconds. Trigeminal neuralgia affects women more often than men, and it's more likely to occur in people who are older than 50. Trigeminal neuralgia symptoms are often triggered by touching areas of the head that are usually unilateral, and within the distribution of the trigeminal nerve; face, teeth, gums, tongue or lips. Attacks may become more frequent and intense over time, and sread over a wider area.[1]

Traditional treatment for Trigeminal neuralgia usually starts with medications, and some people don't need any additional treatment. Doctors usually prescribe carbamazepine for trigeminal neuralgia. Other anticonvulsant drugs that may be used to treat trigeminal neuralgia include oxcarbazepine (Trileptal), lamotrigine (Lamictal) and phenytoin (Dilantin, Phenytek).

However, over time, some people with the condition may stop responding to medications, or they may experience unpleasant side effects. For those people, injections or surgery provide other trigeminal neuralgia treatment options.

Acupuncture has been used for Trigeminal neuralgia with some success, and some reviews find it is as effective as medication, and with less side effects.[2] As most patients are over 50, side effects from medications are often a problem.

A systematic review of 12 studies found that acupuncture is of similar efficacy as carbamezapine, but with fewer adverse effects in treatment of Trigeminal neuralgia.

However, the evidence is weak because of low methodological quality of the reviewed studies.2.

A systematic review and meta-analysis found that manual acupuncture improved the response rate and achieved more significant effect on alleviating pain intensity, and acupuncture combined with carbamazepine had a more positive effect on response rate than carbamazepine alone.[3] The most common points for trigeminal neuralgiaare LI 4, ST 7, GB 20 and Ashi tender points.[4]

References

1. https://www.mayoclinic.org/diseases-conditions/trigeminal-neuralgia/symptoms-causes/syc-20353344

2. Liu H(1), Li H, Xu M, Chung KF, Zhang SP,A systematic review on acupuncture for trigeminal neuralgia, Altern Ther Health Med. 2010 Nov-Dec;16(6):30-5.

3. Hu H(1), Chen L(2), Ma R(2), Gao H(2), Fang J(3).,Acupuncture for primary trigeminal neuralgia: A systematic review and PRISMA-compliant meta-analysis. Complement Ther Clin Pract. 2019 Feb;34:254-267.

4. Tao S, Xu W, Gao Z, Dong Q., Analysis on acupoint selection rule of acupuncture for trigeminal neuralgia, Zhongguo Zhen Jiu. 2016 Feb;36(2):207-11.

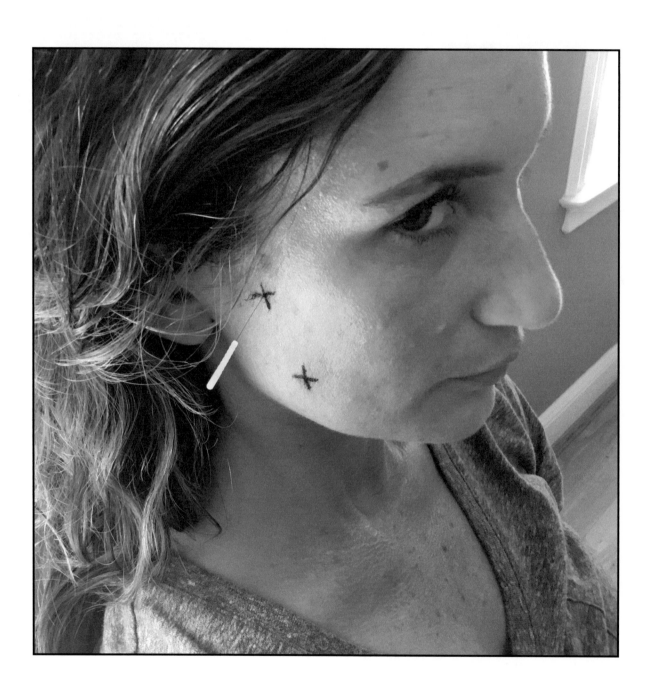

Acupuncture for Bell's Palsy

Bell's palsy is characterised by an acute onset of unilateral, lower motor neuron weakness of the facial nerve in the absence of an identifiable cause. The basic assessment should include a thorough history and physical examination as the diagnosis of Bell's palsy is based on exclusion. For confirmed cases of Bell's palsy, corticosteroids are the mainstay of treatment and should be initiated within 72 hours of symptom onset. Antiviral therapy in combination with corticosteroid therapy may confer a small benefit. Acupuncture has emerged as an alternative therapy for Bell's palsy in both adults and children. However, the use of acupuncture is controversial. A systematic review and meta-analysis to assess the efficacy of acupuncture for Bell's palsy suggested that acupuncture seems to be an effective therapy for Bell's palsy, but there was insufficient evidence to support the efficacy and safety of acupuncture.[1,2]

Incomplete recovery from facial palsy results in social and physical disabilities, and the medical options for the sequelae of Bell's palsy are limited. Acupuncture is widely used for Bell's palsy patients in East Asia, but its efficacy is unclear. A randomized controlled trial including participants with the sequelae of Bell's palsy with the following two parallel arms: an acupuncture group (n = 26) and a waiting list group (n = 13). The acupuncture group exhibited greater improvements in the Facial Disability Index score. Compared with the waiting list group, acupuncture had better therapeutic effects on the social and physical aspects of sequelae of Bell's palsy.[3]

References

1. Phan NT, Panizza B, Wallwork B,A general practice approach to Bell's palsy, Aust Fam Physician. 2016 Nov;45(11):794-797.

2. Li P(1), Qiu T(1), Qin C(1), Efficacy of Acupuncture for Bell's Palsy: A Systematic Review and Meta-Analysis of Randomized Controlled Trials,. PLoS One. 2015 May 14;10(5):e0121880. doi: 10.1371/journal.pone.0121880.eCollection 2015.

3. Kwon HJ(1), Choi JY(2), Lee MS(3), Kim YS(4), Shin BC(5), Kim JI(6),Acupuncture for the sequelae of Bell's palsy: a randomized controlled trial, Trials. 2015 Jun 3;16:246. doi: 10.1186/s13063-015-0777-z..

Acupuncture for Sleep, insomnia

Acupuncture is good for relaxation and has benefits for people with sleep problems. Primary insomnia[1] is defined as a symptom of prolonged sleep latency, difficulties in maintaining sleep, the experience of non-refreshing or poor sleep coupled with impairments of daytime functioning, including reduced alertness, fatigue, exhaustion, dysphoria and other symptoms. The Diagnostic and Statistical Manual of Mental Disorders further defines the condition to be not attributable to a medical, psychiatric or environmental cause. Chronic insomnia (with symptoms at least 3 nights a week for at least 1 month) presents a substantially increased risk for other psychiatric disorders, especially depression, as well as for cardiovascular morbidity and mortality. The prevalence of insomnia disorder is approximately 10–20%, with approximately 50% having a chronic course.[4]

A single-center, single-blinded, and randomized controlled clinical trial of seventy-two patients with primary insomnia, who were randomly assigned into two groups - the acupuncture group, who received acupuncture treatment, and the control group, who received sham acupuncture treatment. The results suggested that acupuncture treatment is more effective than sham acupuncture treatment in increasing insomnia patients' sleep quality and improving their psychological health.[4] There is evidence that acupuncture could be an alternative therapy to medication for treating depression related insomnia. [5,6]

References

1. Fortier-Brochu E, Beaulieu-Bonneau S, Ivers H, *et al*, World Health Organization. *The international statistical classification of diseases and related health*

2. Baglioni C, Battagliese G, Feige B, et al, Insomnia and daytime cognitive performance: a meta-analysis. Sleep Med Rev 2012; 16:83–94. doi:10.1016/j.smrv.2011.03.008

3. Sofi F, Cesari F, Casini A, et al Insomnia as a predictor of depression: a meta-analytic evaluation of longitudinal epidemiological studies. J Affect Disord 2011;135:10–19. doi:10.1016/j.jad.2011.01.011

4. Buysse DJ, Efficacy and safety of acupuncture treatment on primary insomnia: a randomized controlled trial, Insomnia. JAMA 2013;309:706–16. doi:10.1001/jama.2013.193 Sleep Med. 2017 Sep;37:193-200. doi: 10.1016/j.sleep.2017.02.012. Epub 2017 Mar 8.

5. Yin X[1], Gou M[2], Xu J[1], Dong B[1], Yin P[1], Masquelin F[1], Wu J[1], Lao L[3], Xu S[4], A Systematic Review and Meta-Analysis of Acupuncture for treating depression-related insomnia indicated that acupuncture could be an alternative therapy to medication for treating depression-related insomnia.

6. Dong B[1], Chen Z[1], Yin X[1], Li D[2], Ma J[1], Yin P[1], Cao Y[1], Lao L[3], Xu S[1], The Efficacy of Acupuncture for Treating Depression-Related Insomnia Compared with a Control Group: A Systematic Review and Meta-Analysis, Biomed Res Int. 2017;2017:9614810.

Acupuncture for aging and well being

Acupuncture is a system of medicine which developed in Asia over thousands of years and is the oldest continually practiced medicine in the world. Acupuncture is not just the use of needles to reduce pain, but rather is a method of balancing the nervous system and organ systems in the body. There are numerous modern medical theories about how acupuncture works. Acupuncture stimulates the flow of pain-relieving endorphins and opioids, releases neurotransmitters, and has effects on both the autonomic nervous system and the immune system.

Acupuncture has been shown to reduce pain in chronic pain conditions such as myofascial pain, as well as many other pain conditions [1,2]. Differences in fMRI mapping of deactivation/activation of brain hemodynamic patterns were reported between acupuncture treatment and pain/tactile stimulation, and an overlap in hemodynamic patterns between brain at sleep and after a 29 minute stress-reduction acupuncture treatment [3]. During administration of verum acupuncture, fMRI changes were found in the pain centers of the brain; orbitofrontal cortex, insula, and pons while diprenorphine positron emission tomography demonstrated signal changes in the orbitofrontal cortex, medial prefrontal cortex, insula, thalamus, and anterior cingulate cortex [4]. Considering that a lateral network in the brain is associated with the sensory aspects of pain perception while a medial network is associated with affective aspects, the highest concentration of opioid receptors being in the medial network, there is strong evidence that acupuncture analgesia is mediated at least in part by opioid systems [4].

Acupuncture can be a great help for many health problems of aging, as well as helping with prevention and general well-being.

Chronic pain can be a major block for many, affecting mobility, mood and appetite. Many of the drugs used to combat chronic pain result in major side effects, such as impaired cognition, memory, balance, and dry mouth. Acupuncture can be an effective treatment for chronic pain by itself, or used in conjunction with medication, to reduce the dosage and minimize the side effects.

Depression can result from many conditions of aging; loss of friends and family, isolation, decreased energy and stamina. Acupuncture can combat depression by increasing your endorphan levels, and giving you a feeling of well-being, as well as more energy, and better appetite.

Acupuncture has shown some evidence for helping Parkinson's Disease.6 Acupuncture is used as one modality to help improve the quality of life of the elderly.

References

1. La Touche R, Goddard G, De-la-Hoz JL, Wang K, Paris-Ale-many A, Angulo-Díaz-Parreñi S, Mesa J, Hernández M. Acupuncture in the treatment of pain in temporomandibular disorders: A systematic review and meta-analysis of randomized controlled trials. Clin J Pain 2010;26:541-50.

2. Cho SH, Whang WW. Acupuncture for temporomandibular disor-ders: A systematic review. J Orofac Pain 2010;24:152-62.

3. Hui KK, Napadow V, Liu J, Li M, Marina O, Nixon EE, Claunch JD, LaCount L, Sporko T, Kwong KK. Monitoring acupuncture effects on human brain by FMRI. J Vis Exp 2010;38:1190.

4. Dougherty DD, Kong J, Webb M, Bonab AA, Fischman AJ, Gol-lub RL. A Combined [11c] diprenorphine PET Study and fMRI Study of Acupuncture Analgelsia. Behav Brain Res

5. Yin X[1], Gou M[2], Xu J[1], Dong B[1], Yin P[1], Masquelin F[1], Wu J[1], Lao L[3], Xu S[4], A Systematic Review and Meta-Analysis of Acupuncture for treating depression-related insomnia indicated that acupuncture could be an alternative therapy to medication for treating depression-related insomnia.

6. Ko JH, Lee H, Kim SN, Park HJ, Does Acupuncture Protect Dopamine Neurons in Parkinson's Disease Rodent Model?: A Systematic Review and Meta-Analysis.,Front Aging Neurosci. 2019 May 8;

7. Van Rijckevorsel-Scheele J, Willems RCWJ, Roelofs PDDM, Koppelaar E, Gobbens RJJ, Goumans M, Effects of health care interventions on quality of life among frail elderly: a systematized review.,Clin Interv Aging. 2019 Apr 4;14:643-658.

8. Acupuncture and Placebo

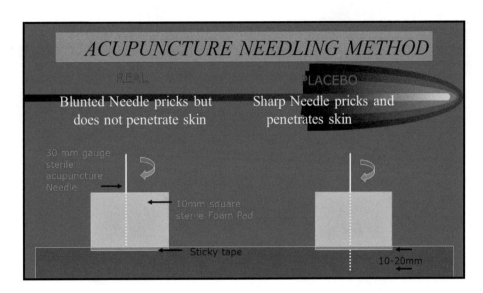

Does acupuncture work as a placebo? The construct behind placebo effect and meaning response have changed dramatically over the years, especially in more recent years. This has occurred originally as a result of very sophisticated experimental protocols using placebos in clinical studies of patients in pain, as well as various studies involving different kind of diseases like Parkinson's or even in non-clinical settings (sports and doping). [1]

Our understanding of the biological and psychological mechanisms underlying placebo effects has expanded significantly due to recent developments in the technology of brain imaging. Based on findings from brain-imaging analyses, we now know that placebo analgesia is definitely a real (ie, biologically measurable) phenomenon. It can be pharmacologically blocked and behaviorally enhanced, and these responses have been demonstrated to be similar to those elicited by administration of "real" analgesic substances. [2]

Psychological mechanisms involved in placebo analgesia include expectancy, meaning response, and classical conditioning. [3-5]

Modern science now understands that there is a placebo effect in all treatments, and acupuncture also has built in the procedure many powerful actions that make up a placebo effect. In addition to the confidence and caring of the acupuncturist, the placing of needles into the body with minimal pain, enhances the patients experience and expectation of the patient. The feeling of the Chi response and the acupuncturist's positive reaction also has an added effect. Not least is that acupuncture is somewhat foreign to western culture and it might be perceived as magical or spiritual; and this also makes for a positive effect. [6]

Clearly, culture and expectancy are two issues that need to be evaluated in acupuncture studies. It has been argued that acupuncture therapy is different from most Western medical treatments because it views the patient in a holistic way. Viewing the patient "holistically" is associated with a medical philosophy originating from certain Asian cultures. Therefore, "Western" therapeutic research using placebo controls may undermine a large part of the effectiveness of acupuncture. There are problems with double blinding, as it is impossible for the acupuncturist not to know which subject is receiving "real" or sham acupuncture. It is also difficult for subjects to be blinded, especially if they have had acupuncture previously and can recognize the feeling of acupuncture needles penetrating their skin.[7] Efforts are ongoing in order to overcome this point, and creating true 'sham' acupuncture models [7-9]

Acupuncture clearly affects a complex psychophysiological matrix that is intimately intertwined with expectation in both a specific and non-specific manner that is consistent with its specific clinical effects, as well as the effects of expectation on pain relief. From a cultural standpoint, these studies suggest that for a treatment such as acupuncture to be effective, even if it comes from a culture different from that of the provider/patient, a common cultural layer/background must exist, allowing both the provider and the patient to share a common set of expectations or beliefs. Beliefs/expectations are, of course, pre-existing mental/brain states and their top-down non-specific influence on pain experience is well known.

In other terms, it helps that one expects that acupuncture works. But this is generally true for any treatment, drug or procedure

As stated in the introduction, there is no need to adopt any esoteric confession to accept the results of acupuncture in some conditions. For the un-believer, acupuncture can thus be considered at the very least, an elegant type of placebo, similar in many ways to occlusal appliances. It appears that both real and placebo acupuncture can produce significant pain relief for many people.

Acupuncture and splint therapy can be good examples of powerful placebos in the field of TMD. Present knowledge suggests that every treatment for pain contains a placebo component, which sometimes is as powerful as the so-called "active" counterpart. While the deceptive use of placebos must be considered unethical, every health provider who is treating pain patients must be aware of this important phenomenon in order to harness placebo's huge Therefore it should be viewed as a low-risk and high-prudence procedure,[10,11] for successfully and safely treating various types of pain patients.

References

1. Benedetti F. Placebo and the new physiology of the doctor-patient relationship. Physiol Rev. 2013 Jul;93(3)

2. Tétreault P, Mansour A, Vachon-Presseau E, Schnitzer TJ, Apkarian AV, Baliki MN. Brain Connectivity Predicts Placebo Response across Chronic Pain Clinical Trials. PLoS Biol. 2016 Oct 27;14(10)

3. Kaptchuk TJ, Eisenberg DM. The persuasive appeal of alternative medicine. Ann Intern Med 1998;129: 1061–1065.

4. Kaptchuk TJ. Powerful placebo: The dark side of the randomised controlled trial. Lancet 1998;351:1722–1725.

5. Beecher HK. The powerful placebo. JAMA 1955;159:1602–1606.

6. Lao L, Bergman S, Hamilton GR, Langenberg P, Berman B, Evaluation of acupuncture for pain control after oral surgery: a placebo-controlled trial, Arch Otolaryngol Head Neck Surg. 1999 May;125(5):567-72.)

7. Goddard G, Karibe H, McNeill C, Villafuerte E, Acupuncture and sham acupuncture reduce muscle pain in myofascial pain patients,J Orofac Pain. 2002 Winter;16(1):71-6.

8. Park J, White A, Stevinson C, et al. Validating a new non-penetrating sham acupuncture device: two randomized controlled trials. Acupunct Med 2002;20:168–74.)

9. Goddard G, Shen Y, Steele B, Springer N, A controlled trial of placebo versus real acupuncture, J Pain. 2005 Apr;6(4):237-42.

10. Greene CS, Goddard G, Macaluso GM, Mauro G. Topical review: placebo responses and therapeutic responses. How are they related? J Orofac Pain. 2009 Spring;23(2):93-107

11. Stohler CS, Zarb GA. On the management of temporo- mandibular disorders: A plea for a low-tech, high-prudence therapeutic approach. J Orofac Pain 1999;13:255–261.

PART 2

CLINICAL HANDBOOK

9. Sterilization and infection control

Acupuncture is an invasive procedure that pierces the skin, and as such, basic standards of sterilization and infection control must be undertaken. Infections from needles are very rare.

Most acupuncture needles come in individual unit packages that are pre- sterilized. If not, then needles should be packaged and autoclaved. Use of unsterilized needles runs the risk of transmitting blood-borne pathogens, such as Human Immunovirus and Hepatitis virus from one patient to another. Also, other pathogens that could contaminate the needle, such as Staphylococcus, could be inadvertently introduced into the tissue.

The skin should be prepped with an alcohol wipe to disinfect the area prior to inserting the needle. As with any sterile needle, care must be taken to not touch or let the needle contact anything.

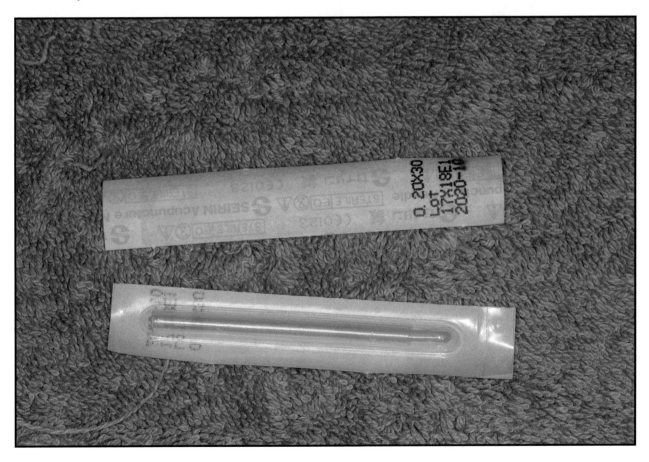

10. Safety, complications

Acupuncture is safe because it is nontoxic and it has minimal adverse reactions, unlike many other conventional treatment modalities. There is no risk of dependency as there is with the use of narcotics. It is simple and convenient if performed by a well-trained practitioner.

The disadvantages of acupuncture are that it is more time consuming, and in many cases, may fail to bring about complete analgesia. It is not suitable for children, because few children will tolerate the needling, and it cannot be used effectively in needle-phobic patients, however the hand often is better than the mouth.

Inadequate insertion of acupuncture needle might cause serious adverse events and tissue injury. Furthermore, the cross-infection of the hepatitis B or HIV is the other threatening adverse effect of using unsterilized needles. However, with increased awareness about the importance using disposable needles, such infections have been mostly eliminated in acupuncture therapy by professional healthcare providers. In a large-scale survey of 2.2 million consecutive acupuncture treatments, adverse events were detected in two patients (pneumothorax and lower limb nerve injury). [1]

Acupuncture is a very safe procedure, with serious complications being very rare. Complications are Pneumothorax, hematoma, bleeding, infection, syncope, pain, broken needle, and feeling of tiredness. However, feelings of relaxation are quite common. [2]

Complications can sometimes be life threatening, such as Pneumothorax. In dental acupuncture, we should not be needling points over the lung, and therefore, this should not be an issue.

Organ damage is rare, but needles should avoid major organs and blood vessels. Care must be exercised when needling near the eyes.

Hematoma can occur when a needle penetrates a blood vessel and bleeding occurs in the tissue. This is rarely serious and an explanation along with a cold compress is all that is usually needed.

Bleeding at the point of entry when the needle is removed, and only needs a gauze compress and explanation. Many acupuncturists count bleeding as a positive sign. Infection is rare, and basic precautions and use of sterile needles will eliminate any chance of infection. Needling should never be performed in areas of active infection, such as an abcess or other infection.

Syncope or fainting can occur, and is managed by placing patient with head down, and comforting until recovery.

Pain is one of the most common complications of needling. Pain is usually from the needle being in a spot that is irritating a nerve ending, and is very uncomfortable, and does not subside after a few seconds. This is very different from the ache or electric shock feeling of De Qi, which calms down after a few seconds. The needle needs to be moved to another area. This can be accomplished by partially withdrawing the needle and re-inserting in a different direction. Sometimes the needle will need to be completely removed from that point.

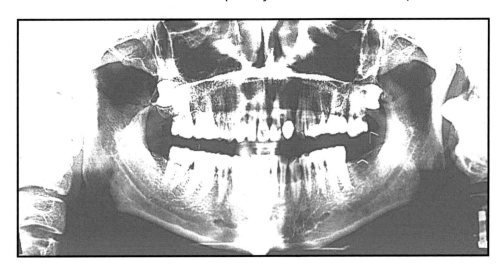

Broken retained acupuncture needles seen on X-ray

Broken needles are very rare, especially since the advent of single us needles that are made of high quality stainless steel and are very flexible. However, a broken needle is always possible, especially if the patient moves and hits the inserted needle.

The feeling of tiredness can be considered a complication, and the patient should rest and avoid any extensive activity for a few hours after acupuncture.

Ernst and White, in their systematic review, found that the incidence of minor adverse events (AEs) associated with acupuncture may be considerable, serious adverse events are rare. The most common adverse events were needle pain (1% to 45%) from treatments, tiredness (2% to 41%), and bleeding (0.03% to 38%). Feelings of faintness and syncope were uncommon, with an incidence of 0% to 0.3%. Feelings of relaxation were reported by as many as 86% of patients. Pneumothorax was rare, occurring only twice in nearly a quarter of a million treatments.[3]

Acupuncture is increasingly used worldwide. It is becoming more accepted by both patients and healthcare providers. However, the current understanding of its adverse events (AEs) is fragmented. Chan, et al. in their systematic reviews (SRs) on the AEs of acupuncture and related therapies, found AEs, which were deaths, organ or tissue injuries, infections, and dizziness or syncope.[4]

Minor and serious AEs can occur during the use of acupuncture and related modalities, contrary to the common impression that acupuncture is harmless. Serious AEs are rare, but need significant attention as mortality can be associated with them. Patient safety should be a core part of acupuncture education.

References

1. Witt CM, Pach D, Brinkhaus B, Wruck K, Tag B, Mank S, et al. Safety of acupuncture: Results of a prospective observational study with 229,230 patients and introduction of a medical information and consent form. Forsch Komplementmed. 2009;16:91–7.

2. Naik PN, Kiran RA, Yalamanchal S, Kumar VA, Goli S, Vashist N. Acupuncture: An Alternative Therapy in Dentistry and Its Possible Applications. Med Acupunct. 2014;26(6):308–314.

3. Ernst E(1), White AR. Prospective studies of the safety of acupuncture: a systematic review. Am J Med. 2001 Apr 15;110(6):481-5.

4. Chan MWC, Wu XY, Wu JCY, Wong SYS, Chung VCH. Safety of Acupuncture: Overview of Systematic Reviews. Sci Rep. 2017 Jun 13;7(1):3369. doi: 10.1038/s41598-017-03272-0

11. Consent

Either verbal or written consent should be obtained before performing acupuncture. Consent should explain that sterile needles will be inserted into points on the body for specific effects, and list the possible complications. See sample consent form below that may be printed and used.

SAMPLE CONSENT FORM INFORMED CONSENT FOR ACUPUNCTURE TREATMENT

I hereby voluntarily consent to receive acupuncture administered by _____, who is qualified to use acupuncture for treatment in dentistry.

I understand that acupuncture is the insertion of sterile needles into points on the body.

I am aware that acupuncture may have occasional unwanted effects (side effects) including bruising, bleeding, fainting, temporary pain or discomfort, and rarely skin infections. I understand that the risk of contracting blood infections such as HIV and Hepatitis is almost non-existent, due to the use of sterile disposable needles.

Treatment has been fully explained to me, my questions have been answered, and I indicate my acceptance by signing below.

Patient _____ Date _____

Doctor _____ Date _____

12. Needling Techniques

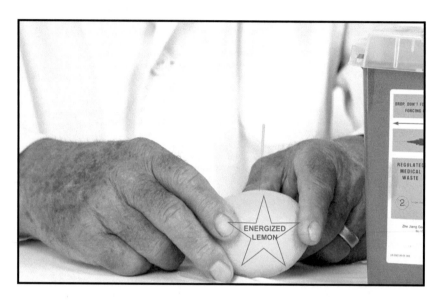

Armamentarium: needles, Needling techniques, tube tapping, finger insertion, lemon, tubes, pecking, rotation, clock and counter, vibration

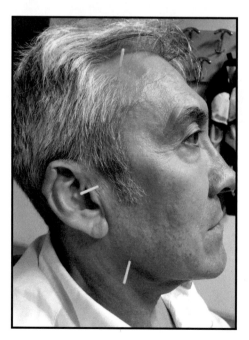

Several types of acupuncture needles are used; they may be small, thin, stainless steel or thick, or even long needles made of silver and gold. Several different types of needles are available, and even dental syringe needles can be used for acupuncture.

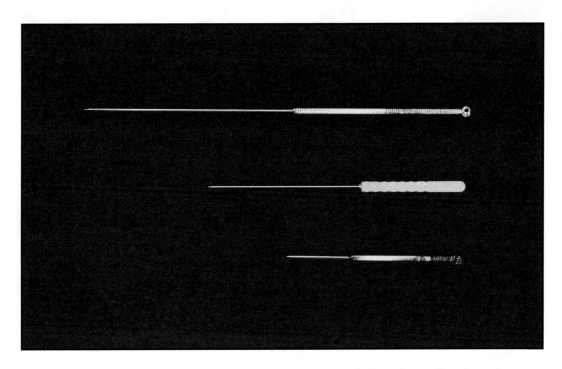

The most common and widely used needles come in individual sterilized packages,, and are contained in a tube to which the handle is attached. The package is opened, the tube with attached needle is removed and placed over the acupuncture point with one hand, held between thumb and forefinger. The handle is then twisted in the tube to detach the handle, and then the forefinger is used to tap the needle through the skin, a few millimeters. The patient should only feel the tap, and not any pain. The tube is then removed and the needle is carefully and slowly inserted with a quarter turn rotating motion until the De Qi response is achieved. The needle can be left in place, typically anywhere from 15 to 30 minutes.

It is common to stimulate the needle once the De Qi is achieved. Usually every five to ten minutes, the needle is stimulated by moving it. The different techniques for stimulation are:

1. Rotation, both clockwise and counter clockwise. The needle is held by the handle with thumb and forefinger, and a quarter turn rotating motion is performed for a few seconds, which often re-stimulates the De Qi.

2. Pecking, which is up and down movement. The needle is held by the handle with thumb and forefinger, and an up and down motion of a few millimeters is performed for a few seconds, and this also often re-stimulates the De Qi.

3. Combination of rotation and pecking. The needle is held by the handle with thumb and forefinger, and an up and down motion, and rotation is performed for a few seconds, and this also often re-stimulates the De Qi.

4. Vibration, running your fingernail up and down the handle sends vibrations into the acupoint and provides a different stimulation that can be beneficial. Flicking the handle with your finger is another technique for stimulation.

5. Other techniques for stimulation of the needles are: heat, often with Moxa over the needle, electrical, hooking the needle up to an electro acupuncture source.

6. Acupuncture points can also be stimulated with acupressure, usually done by the patient after the needles are removed and the patient is dismissed. Patient is instructed to massage one or more points periodically for the next few hours to keep the De Qi flowing.

Video Link:
https://www.youtube.com/watch?v=IfAMuGZ7Ts8&list=PL4NNxK7Mm
T9LMcNRF-o52v0FXuPYdqIZl&index=15&t=0s

The needle is removed by grabbing the handle with thumb and forefinger, and quickly removing with a slight rotation. The needle is then placed in a Sharps container for disposal.

An excellent way to practice needling is the use a piece of fruit; lemons and oranges are good. The skin has a resistance similar to human skin, and one can do hundreds of insertions and removals in a short period. Also stimulation, rotation, pecking, and vibration of the needles can be practiced.

13. TCM measurements

Cun In TCM, every individual is unique, and any measurement is proportional to that person. That is why the Cun is used. A Cun is the width of each persons thumb. A thin person has a smaller width than a big person. If a n acupuncture point, for instance, P6, is located 3 Cuns from the crease in the wrist, it will be proportional to each individual person.

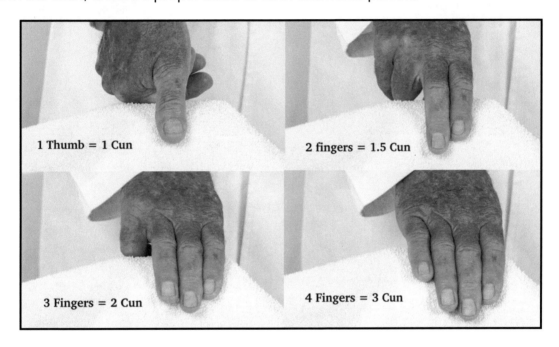

Video Link:
https://www.youtube.com/
watch?v=eX67A_FJRps&list=PL4NNxK7MmT9LMcNRF-
o52v0FXuPYdqlZl&index=13

14. Other Techniques

Moxibustion

Moxibustion therapy consists of burning dried mugwort on particular points on the body. It plays an important role in the traditional medical systems of China, Japan, Korea, Vietnam, and Mongolia. Suppliers usually age the mugwort and grind it up to a fluff; practitioners burn the fluff or process it further into a cigar-shaped stick. They can use it indirectly, with acupuncture needles, or burn it on the patient's skin.[1,2,3]

Theory and practice

Practitioners use moxa to warm regions and meridian points[1,4] with the intention of stimulating circulation through the points and inducing a smoother flow of blood and qi. Some believe it can treat conditions associated with the "cold" or "yang deficiencies" in Chinese Medicine.[5] It is claimed that moxibustion mitigates against cold and dampness in the body, and can serve to turn breech babies.[6,7],8]

Practitioners claim moxibustion to be especially effective in the treatment of chronic problems, "deficient conditions" (weakness), and gerontology. Bian Que (*fl. circa* 500 BCE), one of the most famous semi-legendary doctors of Chinese antiquity and the first specialist in moxibustion, discussed the benefits of moxa over acupuncture in his classic work *Bian Que Neijing*. He asserted that moxa could add new energy to the body and could treat both excess and deficient conditions.

Practitioners may use acupuncture needles made of various materials in combination with moxa, depending on the direction of *qi* flow they wish to stimulate.

There are several methods of moxibustion. Three of them are direct scarring, direct non-scarring, and indirect moxibustion. Direct scarring moxibustion places a small cone of moxa on the skin at an acupuncture point and burns it until the skin blisters, which then scars after it heals.[1,9] Direct non-scarring moxibustion removes the burning moxa before the skin burns enough to scar, unless the burning moxa is left on the skin too long.[1,9] The most practiced technique today is indirect moxibustion that holds a cigar made of moxa near the acupuncture point to heat the skin over the acupuncture point, or holds it on an acupuncture needle inserted in the acupuncture point to heat the needle.[1,9]

There has been very little scientific research into moxibustion. There is a question as to whether the effect of moxibustion is from the moxa, or from the heat energy that is transferred to the acupuncture point. The first modern scientific publication on moxibustion was written by the

Japanese physician Hara Shimetarō who conducted intensive research about the hematological effects of moxibustion in 1927. Two years later his doctoral dissertation on that matter was accepted by the Medical Faculty of the Kyūshū Imperial University.[10] Hara's last publication appeared in 1981.[1, 10]

A Cochrane Review found limited evidence for the use of moxibustion in correcting breech presentation of babies and called for more experimental trials. Side effects included nausea, throat irritation, and abdominal pain from contractions.[11]

References

1. https://en.wikipedia.org/wiki/Moxibustion

2. Huang C, Liang J, Han L, Liu J, Yu M, Zhao B. Moxibustion in early Chinese medicine and its relation to the origin of meridians: a study on the unearthed literatures. Evid Based Complement Alternat Med. 2017;2017:8242136.

3. *Wolfgang Michel (2005). "Far Eastern Medicine in Seventeenth and Early Eighteenth Century Germany". Gengo Bunka Ronkyū 言語文化論究. Kyushu University, Faculty of Languages and Cultures. 67–82. hdl:2324/2878. ISSN 1341-0032.*

4. Wilcox L. Moxibustion: e Power of Mugwort Fire. Boulder, CO: Blue Poppy Press; 2008.

5. Deng H, Shen X. The mechanism of moxibustion: ancient theory and modern research. Evid Based Complement Alternat Med. 2013;2013:379291.

6. *Li Zhaoguo (2013). English Translation of Traditional Chinese Medicine: Theory and Practice. 上海三联书店. p. 11. ISBN 978-7-5426-4084-0.*

7. *Needham, J; Lu GD (2002). Celestial lancets: a history and rationale of acupuncture and moxa. Routledge. pp. 262. ISBN 0-7007-1458-8.*

8. Not all acupuncture points can be used for moxibustion. A few of them are preferred in both classical literature and modern research: Zusanli (ST-36), Dazhui (GV-14).

9. https://www.yinovacenter.com/chinese-medicine/moxibustion/

10. English summary of S. Hara's findings Archived 14 July 2014 at the Wayback Machine

11. *Watanabe, Shinichiro; Hakata, Hiroshi; Matsuo, Takashi; Hara, Hiroshi; Hara, Shimetaro (1981). "Effects of Electronic Moxibustion on Immune Response I". Zen Nihon Shinkyu Gakkai Zasshi. (1): 42–50. doi:10.3777/jjsam.31.42.*

12. *Coyle, M. E.; Smith, C. A.; Peat, B (2012). "Cephalic version by moxibustion for breech presentation". Cochrane Database of Systematic Reviews. (5): CD003928. doi:10.1002/14651858.CD003928.pub3. PMID 22592693.*

Cupping

Cupping is a practice used in traditional medicine in several parts of the world, including China and the Middle East. It involves creating suction on the skin using a glass, ceramic, bamboo, or plastic cup. Negative pressure is created in the cup either by applying a flame to the cup to remove oxygen before placing it on the skin or by attaching a suction device to the cup after it is placed on the skin. In "wet cupping," the skin is pierced, and blood flows into the cup. "Dry cupping" doesn't involve piercing the skin. [1]

- There's been some research on cupping, but most of it is of low quality.
- Cupping may help reduce pain, but the evidence for this isn't very strong.
- There's not enough high-quality research to allow conclusions to be reached about whether cupping is helpful for other conditions. [1]

History

The origin of cupping is unclear. For over 3,000 years, the practice has been typically performed unsupervised, by individuals without any medical background. Iranian traditional medicine uses wet-cupping practices, with the belief that cupping with scarification may eliminate scar tissue, and cupping without scarification would cleanse the body through the organs. Individuals with a profound interest in the practice are typically very religious and seek "purification."[2]

There is reason to believe the practice dates from as early as 3000 BC. The Ebers Papyrus, written c. 1550 BC and one of the oldest medical textbooks in the Western world, describes the Egyptians' use of cupping, while mentioning similar practices employed by Saharan peoples. In ancient Greece, Hippocrates (c. 400 BC) used cupping for internal disease and structural problems. The method was highly recommended by Muhammad and hence well-practiced by Muslim scientists who elaborated and developed the method further. Consecutively, this method in its multiple forms spread into medicine throughout Asian and European civilizations. In China, the earliest use of cupping that is recorded is from the famous Taoist alchemist and herbalist, Ge Hong (281–341 A.D.). Cupping was also mentioned in Maimonides' book on health and was used within the Eastern European Jewish community.[2]

As of 2012 cupping was most popular in China. Cupping has been a formal modality in Chinese hospitals since 1950. There is yet much good evidence for the use of cupping. A trial on cupping for fibromyagia showed cupping therapy is more effective for patients with the fibromyalgia syndrome than usual care, but not compared to sham cupping indicating that the effects of cupping therapy might be confounded by unspecific effects.[3]

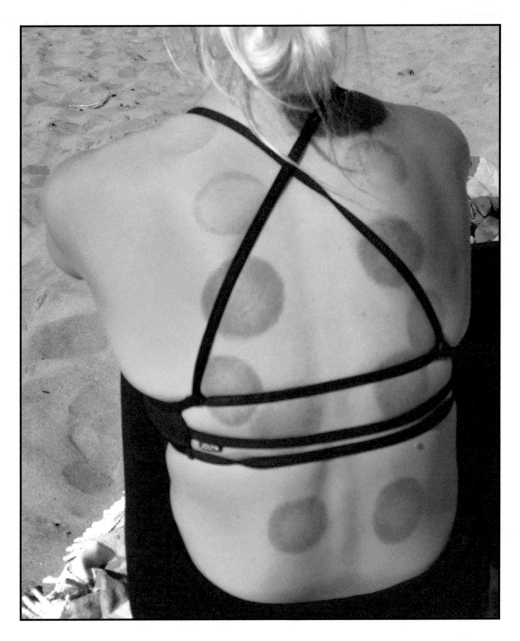

References

1. https://nccih.nih.gov/health/cupping

2. https://en.wikipedia.org/wiki/Cupping_therapy#History

3. Lauche R, Spitzer J, Schwahn B, Ostermann T, Bernardy K, Cramer H, Dobos G, Langhorst J. Efficacy of cupping therapy in patients with the fibromyalgia syndrome-a randomised placebo controlled trial. Sci Rep. 2016 Nov 17;6:37316.

PART 3

DENTAL ACUPUNCTURE POINTS AND INDICATIONS

1. Acupuncture treatment plan: Point selection. Local. Distal. Ashi. Segmental or Central

An acupuncture treatment plan must include a good history, including past medical history, an extensive examination with special attention to painful joints, nerve abnormalities, tender points found in muscle palpation, with attention to any distant pain referral. After all this information is gathered, a good diagnosis can be made, and based on this diagnosis, an acupuncture treatment plan can be developed.

The individualized diagnosis based acupuncture treatment plan should select one or more distal points to draw the pain away. Distal points have more of a central nervous system effect.

Then local points in the area of the patients complaint will be chosen, based on those points that are tender, which are often Ashi points. Local points have more of a segmental effect, as well as a local trigger point effect.

Then, auxillary points based on the patient's condition, will be chosen to reduce stress, anxiety, or give a general feeling of well-being.

For example, a patient diagnosed with myofascial pain of the masticatory muscles and anxiety might have acupuncture needles placed in the distal points of LI 4 and ST 36 to draw the pain away. Then local points such as ST 6 and any other tender Ashi points in the masseter and temporalis muscles will be needled. GV 20 can then be used to give a calming of anxiety and general well-being.

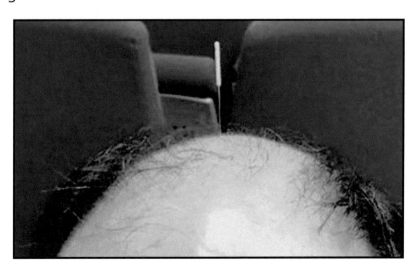

2. Dental Acupuncture Points and Indications.

LI-4, Large Intestine 4, Hegu, Hoku

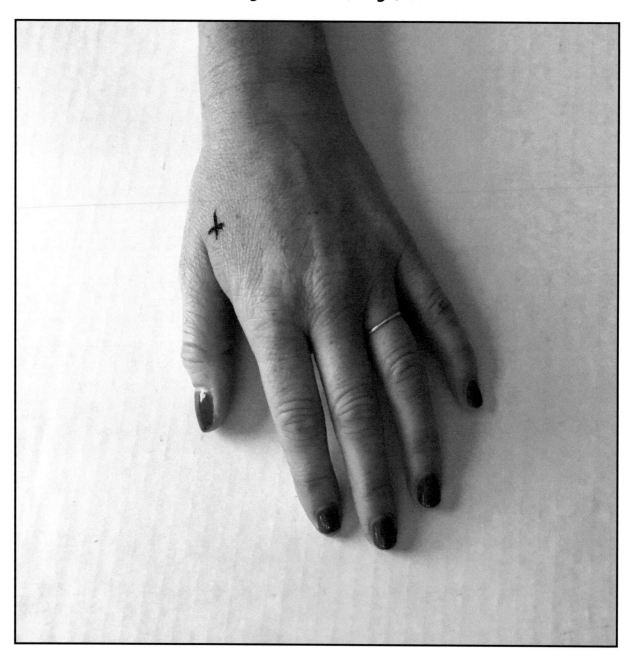

Location: On the dorsum of the hand between the 1st and 2nd metacarpal bones, slightly to the index finger side. the thumb and forefinger together, go up the crease between the two, then to the top of the medial adductor pollicis muscle towards the index finger.

Needling technique: perpendicular insertion, 10 to 20 mm.

Caution: Not to be used in pregnant women.

Indications: LI-4 is the most important analgesic point, most frequently used point, and stimulation of this point relieves pain in all parts of the body. It is especially important for dental and orofacial pain. It is used for tooth pain, jaw/face pain and headache. It also has a strong relaxation effect, probably due to endorphin release.

- INDICATIONS; TMD PAIN, TMJ SYNOVITIS, TMJ OSTEOARTHRITIS, MYOFASCIAL PAIN, FIBROMYALGIA, NEUROPATHIC PAIN, NECK PAIN, HEADACHE, TENSION AND MIGRAINE, TOOTH ACHE, ANALGESIA OF MOUTH, DRY MOUTH, BURNING MOUTH and TONGUE, TINNITIS, and RELAXATION.

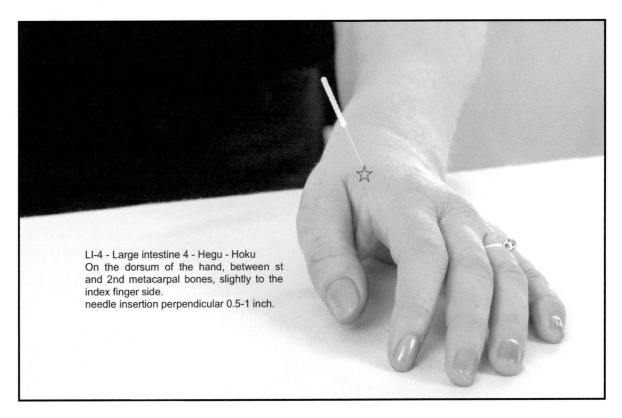

LI-4 - Large intestine 4 - Hegu - Hoku
On the dorsum of the hand, between st and 2nd metacarpal bones, slightly to the index finger side.
needle insertion perpendicular 0.5-1 inch.

Video Link:
 https://www.youtube.com/watch?v=u9TzAlzZ-Hc&list=PL4NNxK7MmT9LMcNRF-o52v0FXuPYdqIZl&index=11

ST-36, Stomach 36, Zusanli

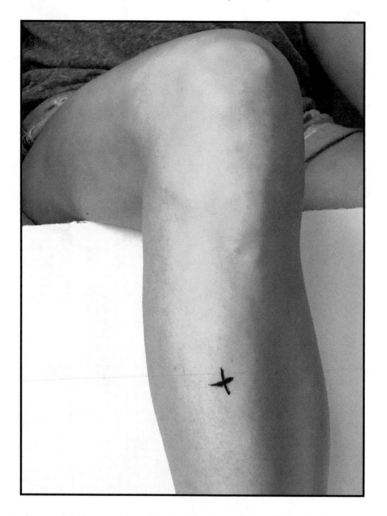

Location: One finger's breadth lateral to the lower border of the tuberositas tibae, 3 cun below the knee joint. If one runs the finger down the lateral side of the tibia, there usually will be a depression about 3 cuns below the knee, and the depression is the point.

Needling technique: perpendicular insertion, 20 to 30 mm.

Indications: ST-36 is one of the most important distal analgesic points, used for pain, analgesia, neuropathic pain, and nausea and vomiting.

- INDICATIONS; TMD PAIN, TMJ SYNOVITIS, TMJ OSTEOARTHRITIS, MYOFASCIAL PAIN, FIBROMYALGIA, NECK PAIN, HEADACHE, TENSION AND MIGRAINE, NEUROPATHIC PAIN, TOOTH ACHE, ANALGESIA OF MOUTH, DRY MOUTH, BURNING MOUTH/ TONGUE, TINNITIS.

   Video Link:
   https://www.youtube.com/watch?v=lLqVzuR9Hic&list=PL4NNxK7MmT 9LMcNRF-o52v0FXuPYdqlZl&index=10

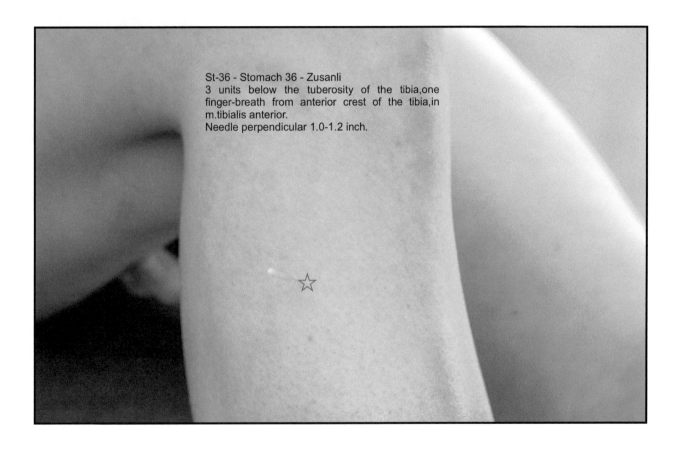

St-36 - Stomach 36 - Zusanli
3 units below the tuberosity of the tibia,one
finger-breath from anterior crest of the tibia,in
m.tibialis anterior.
Needle perpendicular 1.0-1.2 inch.

ST-44, Stomach 44, Neitling

Location: Proximal to the web (about 0.5 cun) between the second and third toes. It is between the second and third metatarsal bones.

Needling technique: perpendicular insertion, 20 to 30 mm, or can be angled towards the ankle.

Indications: ST-44 is an important distal analgesic points, used for dental pain, analgesia, and neuropathic pain.

- INDICATIONS; TMD PAIN, TMJ SYNOVITIS, TMJ OSTEOARTHRITIS, MYOFASCIAL PAIN, FIBROMYALGIA, NEUROPATHIC PAIN, NECK PAIN, HEADACHE, TENSION AND MIGRAINE, TOOTH ACHE, ANALGESIA OF MOUTH, DRY MOUTH, BURNING MOUTH/ TONGUE, and TINNITIS.

    Video Link:
    https://www.youtube.com/watch?v=wnyMNDgBTio&list=PL4NNxK7M
    mT9LMcNRF-o52v0FXuPYdqlZl&index=9

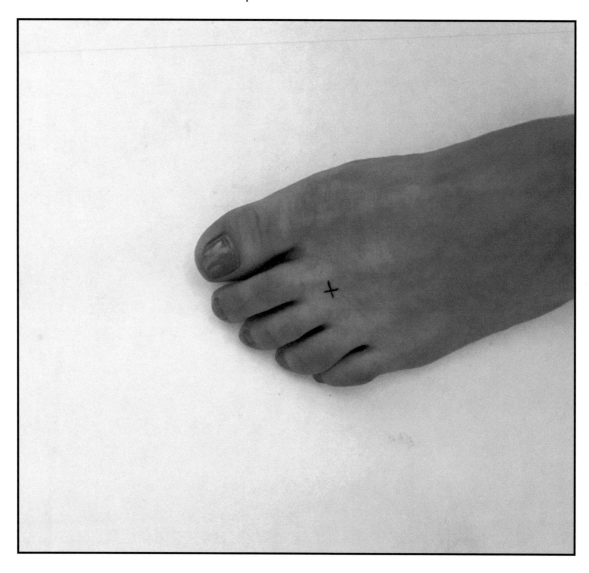

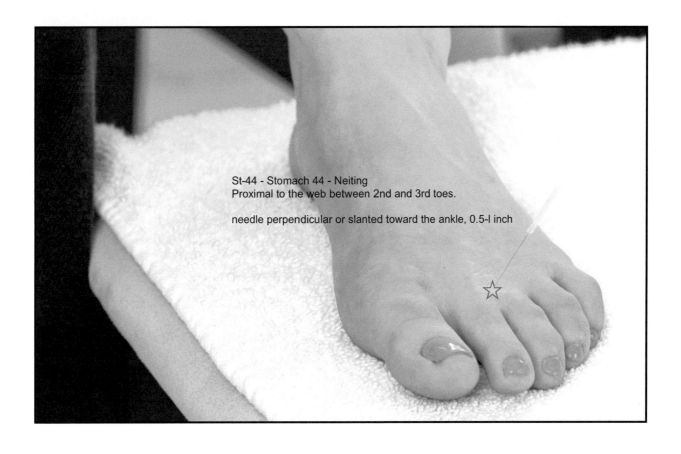

St-44 - Stomach 44 - Neiting
Proximal to the web between 2nd and 3rd toes.

needle perpendicular or slanted toward the ankle, 0.5-l inch

Liv-3, Liver-3, Taichong

Location: On the dorsum of the foot in the depression between the first and second metatarsal bones, 2 cun proximal to the margin of the web.

Needling technique: perpendicular insertion, 10 to 20 mm.

Indications: Liv-3 is good for stress and anxiety, as well as headaches, especially Migraines. It is often used in conjunction with LI-4 for added benefit.

- INDICATIONS; TMD PAIN, TMJ SYNOVITIS, TMJ OSTEOARTHRITIS, MYOFASCIAL PAIN,

   Video Link:
   https://www.youtube.com/watch?v=sQS7kTZozqM&list=PL4NNxK7M
   mT9LMcNRF-o52v0FXuPYdqlZl&index=8

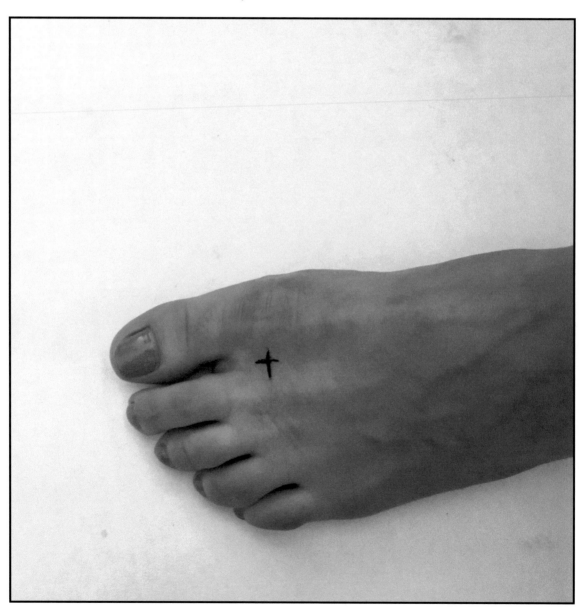

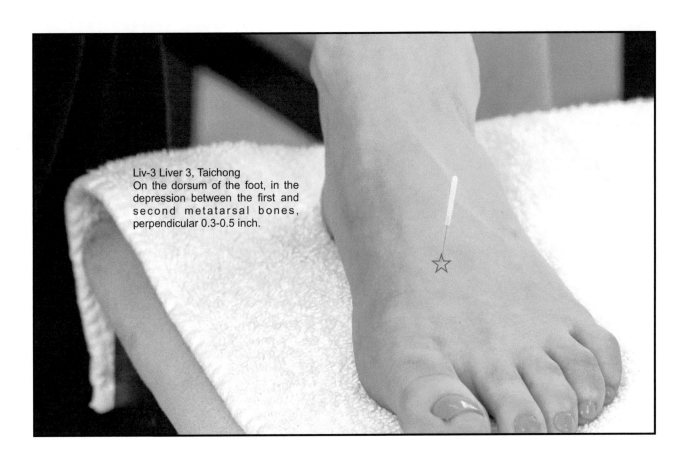

Liv-3 Liver 3, Taichong
On the dorsum of the foot, in the depression between the first and second metatarsal bones, perpendicular 0.3-0.5 inch.

P-6, Pericardium 6, Neiguan.

Location: 2 cun above the transverse crease in the wrist between the two tendons, palmaris longis and flexor radialis.

Needling technique: perpendicular insertion, 10 to 20 mm.

Caution: Avoid tendons and blood vessels in the area.

Indications: P-6 is an important point for gagging during dental procedures, and also is used for treatment of irritability, restlessness, agitation and insomnia.

- INDICATIONS; ANXIETY, DEPRESSION, GAGGING, NAUSEA, BRUXISM
- MOTION SICKNESS, SEA SICKNESS

Video Link:
https://www.youtube.com/watch?v=24PThRbF2HY&list=PL4NNxK7Mm T9LMcNRF-o52v0FXuPYdqlZl&index=7

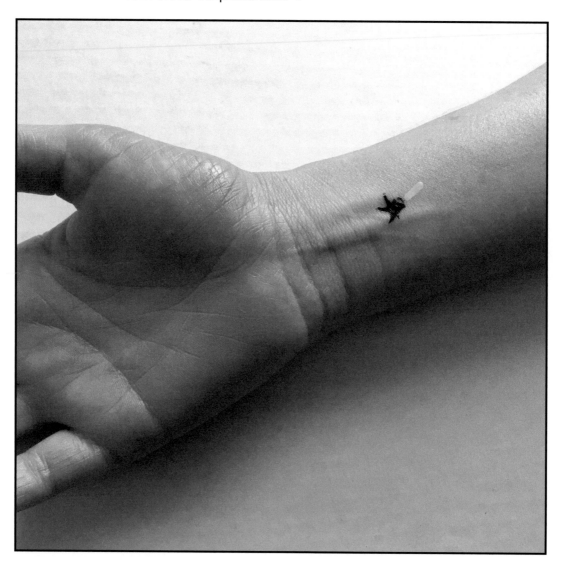

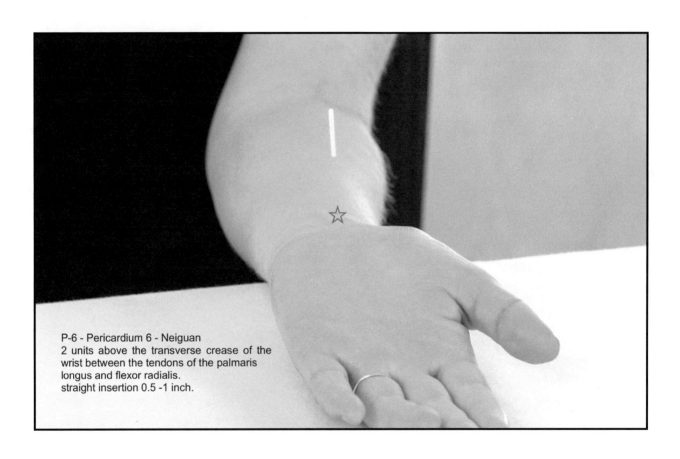

P-6 - Pericardium 6 - Neiguan
2 units above the transverse crease of the wrist between the tendons of the palmaris longus and flexor radialis.
straight insertion 0.5 -1 inch.

Ren-24, Ren Mai 24

Location: In the midline, at the crease between the chin and lip.

Needling technique: perpendicular insertion, 10 to 15 mm.

Indications: Ren-24 has been used with success for gagging, and helps with dry mouth.

- GAGGING
- DRY MOUTH

Video Link:
https://www.youtube.com/watch?v=5poeM8TJmzw&list=PL4NNxK7M
mT9LMcNRF-o52v0FXuPYdqIZl&index=6

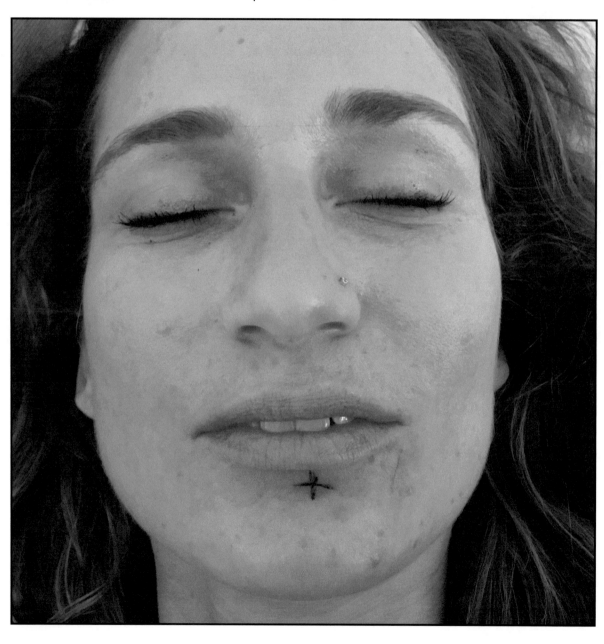

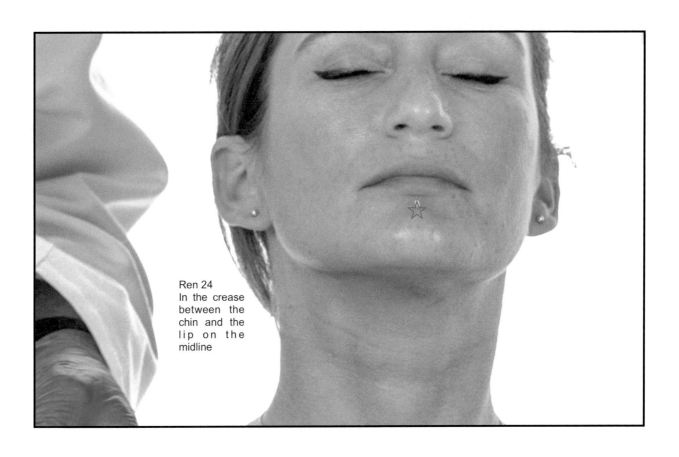

Ren 24
In the crease
between the
chin and the
lip on the
midline

ST-6, Stomach 6, Jiache

Location: At the midpoint of the masseter muscle, when the jaw is closed. One finger breadth anterior and superior to the lower angle of the mandible in the prominence of the masseter muscle when teeth are clenched.

Needling technique: perpendicular insertion, 10 to 25 mm.

Indications: St-6 is the main point in treating myofascial pain of the masticatory muscles, it can also be used in all temporomandibular disorders, and headaches, both tension type and migraine.

- INDICATIONS; TMD'S, TMJ SYNOVITIS, TMJ ARTHRITIS.
- MYOFASCIAL PAIN, FIBROMYALGIA.
- HEADACHE, TENSION AND MIGRAINE.
- TINNITUS

Video Link:
https://www.youtube.com/watch?v=zjPAXnvG1lw&list=PL4NNxK7MmT9LMcNRF-o52v0FXuPYdqIZl&index=5

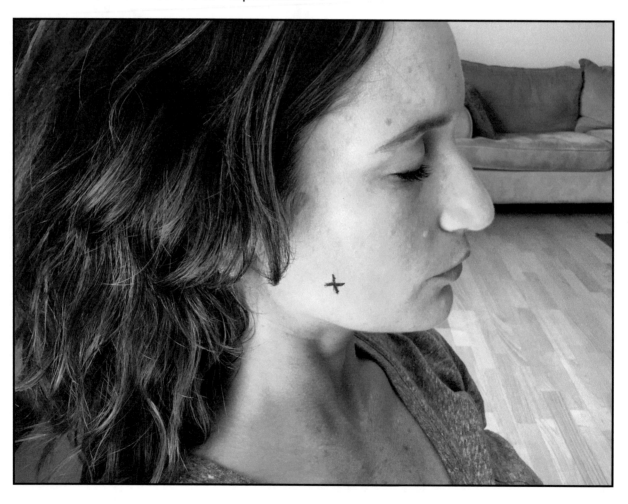

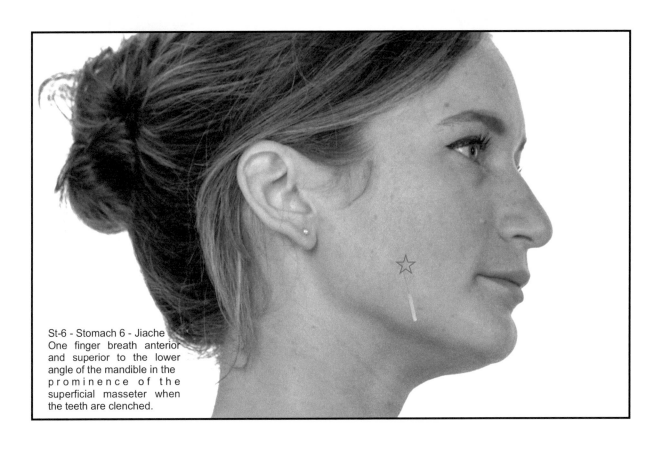

St-6 - Stomach 6 - Jiache
One finger breath anterior
and superior to the lower
angle of the mandible in the
prominence of the
superficial masseter when
the teeth are clenched.

ST-7, Stomach 7, Xiaguan

Location: With the mouth closed, in the depression between the zygpmatic arch and the mandibular arch. If patient opens, palpate the condyle, and the point is in the depression left when the mouth is closed. It is over the deep masseter muscle.

Needling technique: perpendicular insertion, 10 to 25 mm.

Indications: St-7 is the main point in treating temporomandibular joint pain, it can also be used in all temporomandibular disorders, myofascial pain, and headaches, both tension type and migraine.

- INDICATIONS; TMD'S, TMJ SYNOVITIS, TMJ ARTHRITIS.
- MYOFASCIAL PAIN, FIBROMYALGIA.
- HEADACHE, TENSION AND MIGRAINE.
- TINNITIS

Video Link:
https://www.youtube.com/watch?v=8Wqus6rETEs&list=PL4NNxK7Mm
T9LMcNRF-o52v0FXuPYdqIZl&index=4

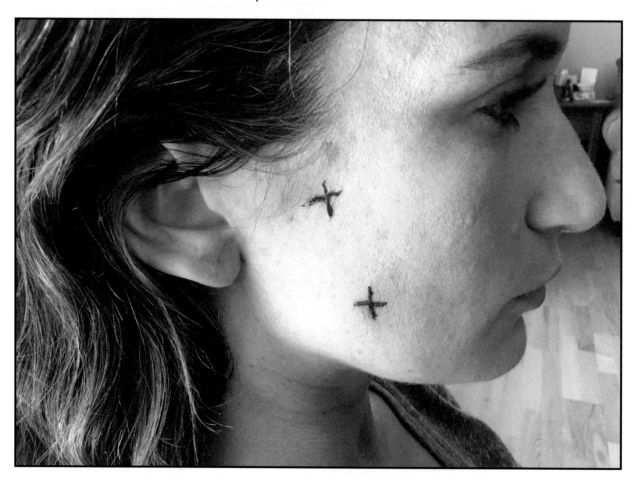

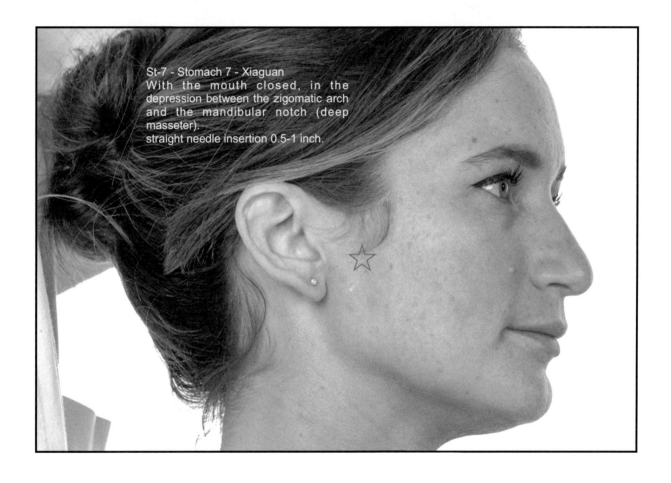

St-7 - Stomach 7 - Xiaguan
With the mouth closed, in the depression between the zigomatic arch and the mandibular notch (deep masseter).
straight needle insertion 0.5-1 inch.

ST-8, Stomach 8, Touwei

Location: 0.5 cun dorsal to the corner of the hairline on the forehead, directly above ST-7. It is 3 cun above the level of the eyebrows. It is located in the anterior temporalis. Needling technique: perpendicular insertion, 10 to 25 mm.

Indications: St-8 is the main point in treating temporomandibular joint pain, it can also be used in all temporomandibular disorders, myofascial pain, and headaches, both tension type and migraine.

- INDICATIONS; MYOFASCIAL PAIN, FIBROMYALGIA.
- HEADACHE, TENSION AND MIGRAINE.
- TINNITIS

Video Link:
https://www.youtube.com/watch?v=c1HRy1QOx_Y&list=PL4NNxK7Mm
T9LMcNRF-o52v0FXuPYdqlZl&index=3

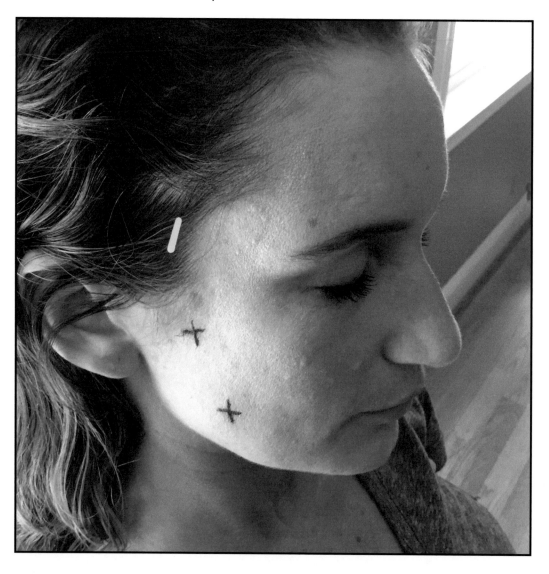

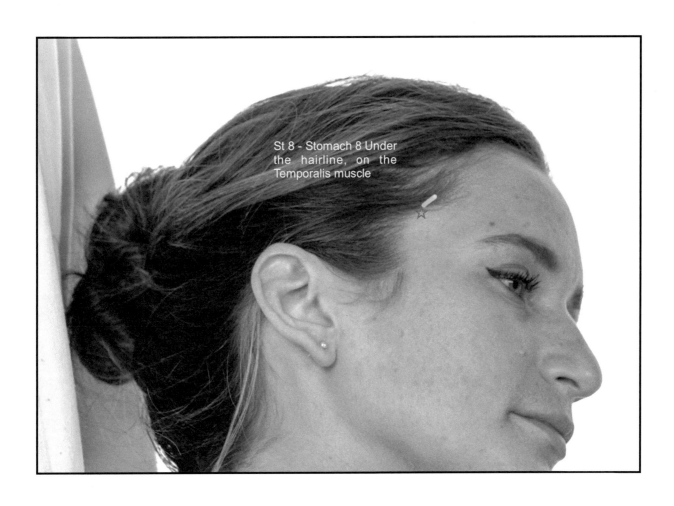

St 8 - Stomach 8 Under the hairline, on the Temporalis muscle

GB-12, Gall Bladder 12, Wangu

Location: On the anterior part of the mastoid process, 1 cun dorsal to the tragus of the ear.

Needling technique: perpendicular insertion, 10 to 15 mm.

Indications: GB-12 is important to address neck symptoms that are playing a role in temporomandibular joint pain, it can also be used in all temporomandibular disorders, myofascial pain, and headaches, especially tension type and migraine with a cervical component..

- INDICATIONS; MYOFASCIAL PAIN, NECK PAIN, FIBROMYALGIA.
- HEADACHE, OCCIPITAL, TENSION AND MIGRAINE.
- TINNITIS

Video Link:
https://www.youtube.com/watch?v=T_szbFumRzc&list=PL4NNxK7Mm
T9LMcNRF-o52v0FXuPYdqIZl&index=2

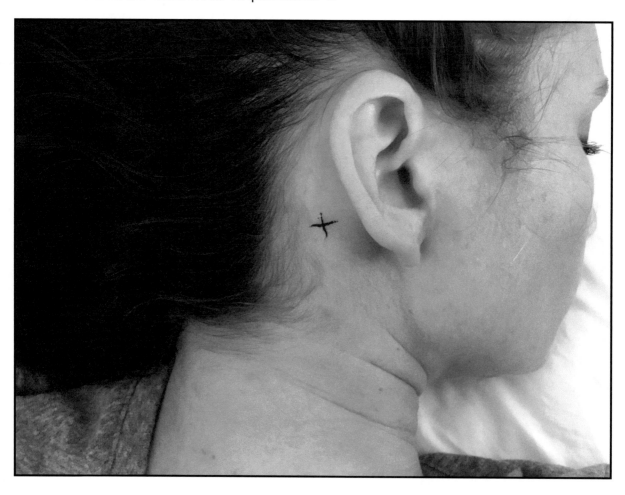

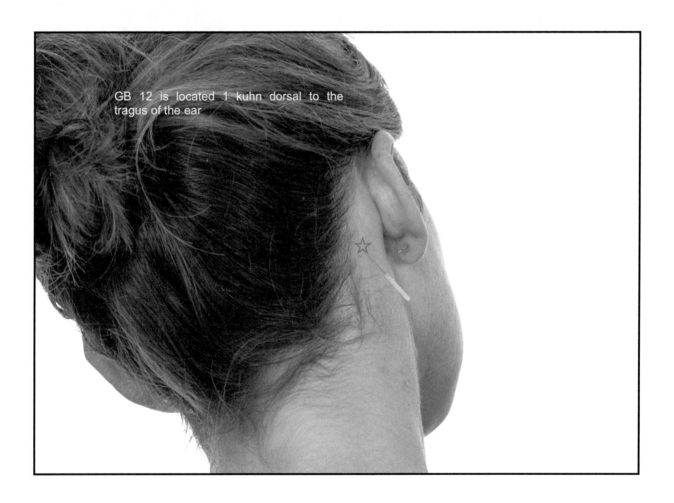

GB 12 is located 1 kuhn dorsal to the tragus of the ear

GB-20, Gall Bladder 20, Fenchi

Location: Between the origins of the sternocleidomastoid and trapezius muscles, and between the occipital bone and the mastoid process.

Needling technique: perpendicular insertion, 10 to 15 mm.

Indications: GB-20 is important to address neck symptoms that are playing a role in temporomandibular joint pain, it can also be used in all temporomandibular disorders, myofascial pain, and headaches, especially tension type and migraine with a cervical component..

- INDICATIONS; MYOFASCIAL PAIN, NECK PAIN, FIBROMYALGIA.

- HEADACHE, OCCIPITAL, TENSION AND MIGRAINE.

- TINNITIS

Video Link:
https://www.youtube.com/watch?v=T_szbFumRzc&list=PL4NNxK7Mm
T9LMcNRF-o52v0FXuPYdqlZl&index=2

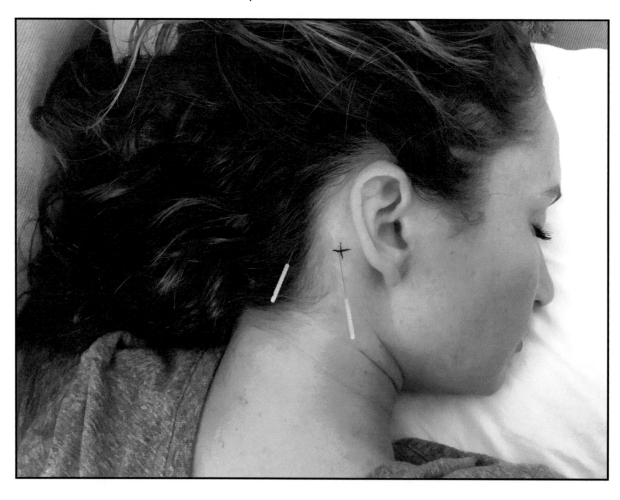

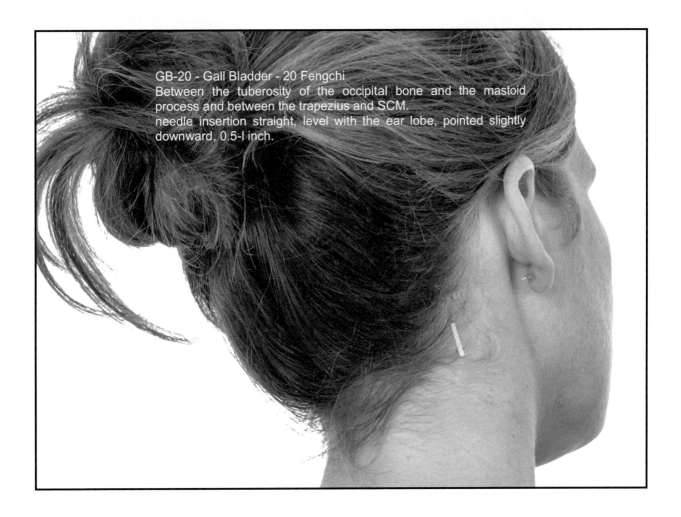

GB-20 - Gall Bladder - 20 Fengchi
Between the tuberosity of the occipital bone and the mastoid
process and between the trapezius and SCM.
needle insertion straight, level with the ear lobe, pointed slightly
downward, 0.5-I inch.

GV-20, Governing Vessel 20, Baihui

Location: On the midline of the head, approximately at the midpoint of the line connecting the lowest and highest points the two ears. At the highest point on the head if one was hanging by a string from that point.

Needling technique: oblique insertion, 5 mm.

Indications: GV-20 is important point that can be used in almost all acupuncture treatments because of its general psychological and harmonizing effect, and the promotion of the feeling of general well-being and relaxation.

- INDICATIONS;TEMPOROMANDIBULAR DISORDERS, MYOFASCIAL PAIN, NECK PAIN, FIBROMYALGIA.
- HEADACHE, OCCIPITAL, TENSION AND MIGRAINE.
- TINNITIS
- GENERAL WELL BEING

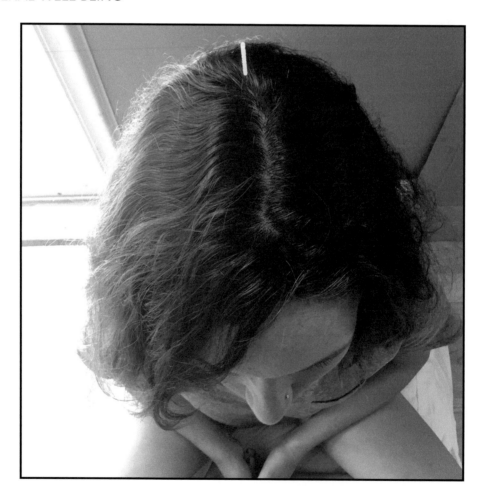

Video Link:
https://www.youtube.com/watch?v=ggUNEt2MEss&list=PL4NNxK7M
mT9LMcNRF-o52v0FXuPYdqIZl&index=1

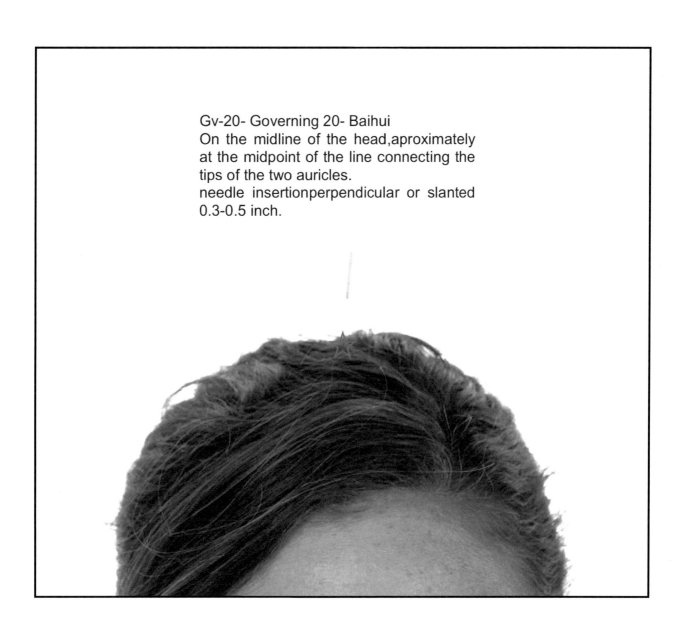

Gv-20- Governing 20- Baihui
On the midline of the head,aproximately
at the midpoint of the line connecting the
tips of the two auricles.
needle insertionperpendicular or slanted
0.3-0.5 inch.

ASHI Points

(Tender points anywhere in a muscle) Also known as trigger points. TCM recommends that Ashi points be a priority in needling, especially when the Ashi points are in the vicinity of the patient's pain complaint. Ashi points often refer pain to distant areas.

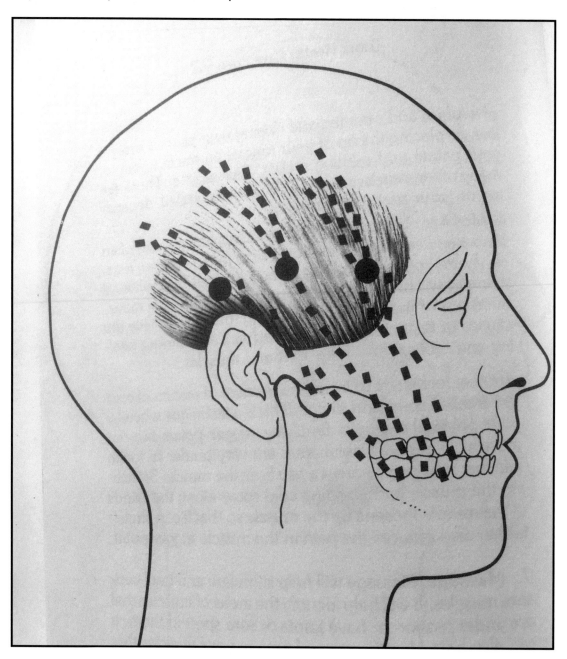

Video Link:
https://www.youtube.com/
watch?v=eX67A_FJRps&list=PL4NNxK7MmT9LMcNRF-
o52v0FXuPYdqIZI&index=13

Location: Found by careful palpation of the affected muscles of the head and neck, and for dentistry and orofacial pain, most commonly the masseter and temporalis, and sternocleidomastoid muscles. Patients may show a withdrawal response when Ashi points are found, and often there is referral of pain to a distant location.

Needling technique: perpendicular insertion, 10 to 25 mm.

Indications: Ashi points are the main points in treating myofascial pain of the masticatory and cervical muscles, and can also be used in all temporomandibular disorders, and headaches, both tension type and migraine.

- INDICATIONS; MYOFASCIAL PAIN, FIBROMYALGIA, HEADACHE, TENSION AND MIGRAINE
- BASIS OF DRY NEEDLING AND TRIGGER POINT THERAPY

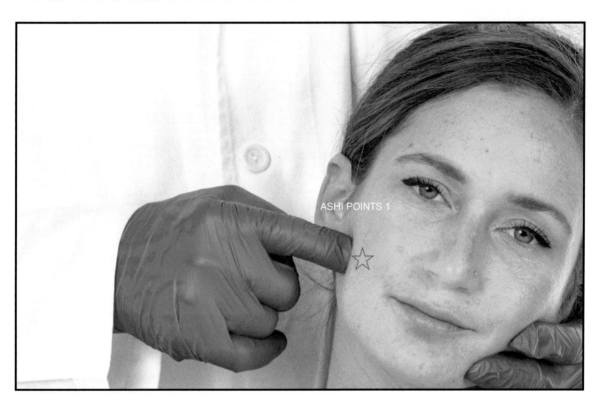

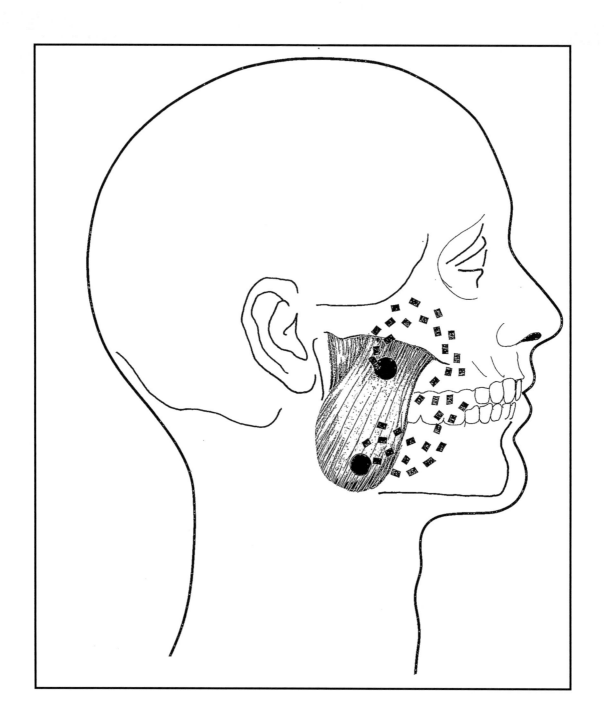

Printed in the United States
by Baker & Taylor Publisher Services